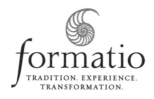

formatio
TRADITION. EXPERIENCE.
TRANSFORMATION.

Formatio books from InterVarsity Press follow the rich tradition of the church in the journey of spiritual formation. These books are not merely about being informed, but about being transformed by Christ and conformed to his image. Formatio stands in InterVarsity Press's evangelical publishing tradition by integrating God's Word with spiritual practice and by prompting readers to move from inward change to outward witness. InterVarsity Press uses the chambered nautilus for Formatio, a symbol of spiritual formation because of its continual spiral journey outward as it moves from its center. We believe that each of us is made with a deep desire to be in God's presence. Formatio books help us to fulfill our deepest desires and to become our true selves in light of God's grace.

ALAN FADLING

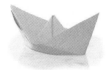

An Unhurried Life

Following Jesus' Rhythms of Work and Rest

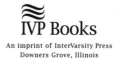

IVP Books

An imprint of InterVarsity Press
Downers Grove, Illinois

InterVarsity Press
P.O. Box 1400, Downers Grove, IL 60515-1426
ivpress.com
email@ivpress.com

InterVarsity Press® is the book-publishing division of InterVarsity Christian Fellowship/USA®, a
movement of students and faculty active on campus at hundreds of universities, colleges and schools of
nursing in the United States of America, and a member movement of the International Fellowship of
Evangelical Students. For information about local and regional activities, visit intervarsity.org.

All Scripture quotations, unless otherwise indicated, are taken from THE HOLY BIBLE, NEW
INTERNATIONAL VERSION®, NIV® Copyright © 1973, 1978, 1984, 2011 by Biblica, Inc.™ Used by
permission. All rights reserved worldwide.

While all stories in this book are true, some names and identifying information in this book have been
changed to protect the privacy of the individuals involved.

Cover design: Cindy Kiple
Interior design: Beth Hagenberg
Images: Hulya Ozkok/Getty Images

ISBN 978-0-8308-3573-7 (print)
ISBN 978-0-8308-8437-7 (digital)

Printed in the United States of America ∞

 As a member of the Green Press Initiative, InterVarsity Press is committed to
protecting the environment and to the responsible use of natural resources. To learn
more, visit greenpressinitiative.org.

Library of Congress Cataloging-in-Publication Data
Fadling, Alan, 1961-
   An unhurried life : following Jesus' rhythms of work and rest / Alan Fadling.
      pages cm
   Includes bibliographical references.
   ISBN 978-0-8308-3573-7 (pbk. : alk. paper)
   1. Time management—Religious aspects—Christianity. 2. Time—Religious aspects—Christianity.
3. Christian life. I. Title.
   BV4598.5.F33 2013
   248.4--dc23

                                                                          2013003935

P	23	22	21	20	19	18	17	16	15	14	13	12	11	10
Y	31	30	29	28	27	26	25	24	23	22	21	20	19	18

Contents

A Frenetic Life

I'm a recovering speed addict—and I don't mean the drug. I'm talking about the inner pace of my life. I always seemed to be in a hurry. I was the guy who looked for the fastest-moving lane on the freeway, the shortest checkout line at the grocery store and the quickest way to finish a job. It's probably pathological. But, like you, I also live in a hurried culture. I'm not the only one trying to get there more quickly and do things faster. In fact, there is little incentive out there to slow down. And the pace in the church doesn't seem all that different from the pace in the world around us.

My journey of recovery, my journey toward a more unhurried life, began when I was in my twenties. At the time I was a full-time college pastor, a full-time student at Fuller Theological Seminary and a new husband. I'm sad to say my priorities were pretty much in that order. I hadn't been in ministry long when a crisis hit. I was convinced that God had invited me to serve his purposes as the focus of my vocational life. But I also knew that I wouldn't be able to continue to do ministry or to live life in the manner or at the pace I had been maintaining. I knew I wouldn't be able to last for many more years or even months, let alone for three or four more decades. My lifestyle was unsustainable. Only in my twenties, I was already showing signs of burnout.

It was at that time that I enrolled in a new Fuller Seminary course titled Collegiate Leadership and Discipleship. My position as a college pastor made the class an obvious choice. While I'm sure I gained many good insights into leading a college ministry, those aren't what I remember. Instead, I remember that built into the course were a couple of daylong retreats that gave me an extended time of solitude and silence with God. The first retreat provoked in me withdrawal-from-busyness symptoms rivaling those of drug addicts during their first week of rehab. I didn't know what to do with myself if I wasn't solving something, going somewhere or helping someone. The hurried pace of my inner life was exposed. There was nothing I could do at the retreat center except listen and no one I could be with except God himself. That retreat marked the beginning of a journey I have now been on for more than twenty years. And I'm still in recovery.

WAS JESUS RELAXED?

As I've traveled this journey, a few words of counsel have guided me. I remember reading what John Ortberg was told during a season of ministry transition in his life: "You must ruthlessly eliminate hurry from your life."[1] Connecting ruthlessness and unhurry has been a fruitful piece of spiritual direction for me. In *The Life You've Always Wanted*, Ortberg suggests that "hurry is not just a disordered schedule. Hurry is a disordered heart."[2] And I agree. When I'm talking about hurried and unhurried, I'm not just talking about miles per hour. I'm talking about an anxious, driven, frenetic heart.

More recently, my friend Bill had a conversation with Dallas Willard,[3] who has mentored many in a lifestyle of spiritual transformation. Dallas asked Bill a simple question: "If you had one word to describe Jesus, what would it be?" What word would you choose? *Teacher? Lord? Compassionate?* Many words would fit. After Bill thought awhile, Dallas offered his own word. It was *relaxed*. Relaxed? Really? That word would not have been on my list. It wasn't on Bill's either. Was it on yours?

Part of me isn't comfortable with the word *relaxed*. It sounds lazy, disengaged, selfish. When Bill told me that story, though, I knew I had to investigate the idea that Jesus was relaxed. What took root in my own heart was the desire to know Jesus as an unhurried Savior. I scheduled for myself a three-day personal retreat and spent the bulk of that time reviewing the Gospels and asking myself over and over, *Was Jesus really relaxed? Was he actually unhurried?*

As the hours became days, it became more and more clear to me that he was definitely more unhurried than the people around him were. After waiting thirty years to begin his ministry, his first ministry act was to follow the Spirit into forty days in the wilderness. His own brothers urged him to do some publicity if he wanted to be a public figure, but Jesus didn't bite (Jn 7:4-6). He seemed frustratingly unhurried on his way to heal the synagogue official's daughter (Mk 5:22-43) and to visit his sick friend Lazarus, who died during Jesus' two-day delay (Jn 11:1-43). His sense of timing often puzzled those around him.

Jesus' unhurried pace also stands in stark contrast to our twenty-first-century pace. Consider, for example, that not many of my friends in vocational ministry waited until they were thirty to get started (Lk 3:23). And to my knowledge, none of them began their ministry with forty days in the wilderness (Lk 4:1-2). The Spirit's leading of Jesus was unhurried. What happened during that wilderness stay? Jesus fasted and he faced temptations orchestrated by the devil. It strikes me that the essence of these temptations was to provoke Jesus to hurry to get for himself what the Father had promised to provide, but in his good timing. I'll talk more about this in chapter four, but it shouldn't come as a surprise to us that a God for whom a day is as a thousand years (2 Pet 3:8) relates to time quite differently than we do!

I believe that modeling our life according to the unhurried pace of Jesus' life and ministry could be a healing and empowering vision for contemporary Christians. Yet many of us measure our faithfulness to God by how many tasks we get done for him or how many meetings we attend to plan his kingdom work. As glad as he is for our service, I believe he is even more pleased when we give him our attention and our friendship.

It seems fitting that I wrote an early draft of this introductory chapter in a quiet room at a retreat center. The setting was idyllic. My window looked out on a long stretch of lawn with trees that seemed to reach up to the heavens in praise. My cell phone coverage dropped out, which I once would have considered a liability but now consider a definite plus. That quiet, unhurried environment exposed my internal struggle with hurry. I feel hurried inside even when nothing actually urgent is on my schedule. Hurry has become a habit: I find myself stuck in emergency mode. Even when nothing outward is pressuring me to pick up the pace, I feel an internal impulse to get to some ill-defined "next thing" that needs my attention. It's pathological. I need healing. I need grace. I need to learn from Jesus himself how to live at his unhurried pace.

The Spirit of God has been working in my heart to teach me how to move at the pace of grace rather than at my own hurried, self-driven pace. I have also realized that an unhurried life is not a lazy life. In fact, it can be the exact opposite.

HOW WE GOT THIS HURRIED

There are a number of reasons why I'm hurried. Maybe some of these same things fuel your hurriedness. First, I've learned, and perhaps I've even been trained, that the faster I go, the more things

I get done. There's some truth to that, of course. But I wonder if all those things I'm getting done matter as much to God—or even to me—as I assume they do. I may be getting more tasks done at a faster pace, but my sense of why I'm doing them has faded. I'm also aware that God's great commandment to us isn't "Get more things done," but to love him with the whole of our energies, capacities and passions and to extend that love to others. And love isn't rushed. The first trait Paul mentioned when he described love in that famous chapter of his is *patient* (see 1 Cor 13). Patience is an unhurried virtue, and it's one of the virtues we have the hardest time with. In my preoccupation with efficiency, I miss much that God wants to do in my life and say to me in the moment. Hurry rushes toward the destination and fails to enjoy the journey.

Adding to the addiction to speed are cultural assumptions about hurry that are built into our mindset. We have a bias toward hurry. Ours is a culture that values speed, efficiency and quickness. Waiting is bad. Getting what we want now is good. Period. We don't stop to ask if what we're getting is even what we most deeply desire. Hurry is a way of life in which advertisers have been mentoring us for years!

This bent toward speed is supported by our very language. Just take a minute to look up the word *slow* in your dictionary. Notice how many of the definitions are negative in tone. My Microsoft Word dictionary offers the following as the first three meanings for the adjective *slow*: "sluggish," "time-consuming" and "stupid." *Merriam-Webster* offers more than a dozen definitions of *slow*. Half are negative, and half are neutral; only one feels positive: "not hasty." The definitions offered for *fast* are far more positive in tone.

Now consider the connection between hurry and boredom. Do you realize that boredom is a modern phenomenon? It's a way of describing how the empty spaces between our hurried activities feel to us. I grew up in a semirural suburb of Sacramento, California, in the 1960s, and what my kids call boring today was the normal pace of my life. Video games, DVDs, cell phones and the like had not become ever-present. We had just three network channels, one PBS channel and one or two local channels on our small TV. Cartoons were a Saturday morning treat; they weren't available 24/7.

Being unhurried doesn't mean being lazy, uninvolved, casual or careless. Those four words expose our culture's false thinking: "Hurry is efficient. Hurry is productive. Hurry is evidence of my importance." Consider the answer we get when we ask, "How are you?" More often than not, the response is "Busy." Although the word is often said with exasperation or resignation, I think just under the surface we believe that we'd be judged as substandard if we ever said, "I have just enough to do," or "These days my yoke is easy and my burden is light." We assume that others will admire our busy and (implied) successful lives. Yet I'm less and less impressed with the outcome of a hurried life. In the long run, does hurry really lead to a fruitful life?

TECHNOLOGY AND SPEED

Since the 1960s and 1970s, our hurry has also been fueled, ironically, by technologies that promise to increase leisure time and give us a much more unhurried existence. Instead, technology has accelerated our pace of life, making our days fuller and giving us much less downtime. We now have the ability to fit more and more tasks into a given amount of time. We have technology to fill every minute with more and more work and activity. We fail to realize how weary and distracted this filled-to-the-brim life makes us. We can get more things done than ever before, but few people would argue that this has made life more meaningful. In fact, a whole new science has emerged that addresses time pathologies. There is time pressure. Time urgency. Most severe is hurry sickness.[4]

Now I don't want to imply that hurry is only a contemporary

issue. Percy Ainsworth, a pastor from the 1800s, said:

> This busy world will surge about you with the tread of restless feet and the throb of restless hearts. And little that you will do will seem to make a pause in the rush of things. But you may in Christ find rest for your soul. You will rest in your work, knowing that duty is eternal; rest in your service of others, knowing that sacrifice is eternal; rest in your purest earthly communion, knowing that love is eternal. This is the hasteless life, and those that "believeth in Christ" will live it.[5]

Where Ainsworth says *hasteless*, I want to suggest *unhurried*. The unhurried life Ainsworth described is what I want. Like me, he longed for a life with rest rather than rush, and he died in 1909! Hurry was just as much a reality one hundred years ago as it is today. We now have technology, though, that enables us to hurry at greater and greater speeds. We can drive five hundred miles or fly five thousand miles today in the same amount of time someone a hundred years ago would have traveled just twenty miles. No wonder hurry is a big issue for us. Our technological tools translate our inward hurry into outward hurry.

I'm not ungrateful for the gift of speed as it relates to technology and transportation. I don't want to access the Internet at dial-up modem speed. I don't want to ride a horse and buggy five hundred miles to visit my extended family. And I'm grateful for a plane that enables me to leave for and arrive in another part of the world on the same day as opposed to weeks- and months-long train trips or ocean voyages.

WANG MINGDAO: WALKING WITH GOD WITHOUT HURRY

In his book, *Faith That Endures*, Ronald Boyd-MacMillan tells the story of a number of conversations he has had with Wang Mingdao, one of China's most famous church pastors of the last century.[6] The first time he met this famous—and persecuted—Chinese pastor, they had the following interchange: "'Young man, how do you walk with God?' I listed off a set of disciplines such as Bible study and prayer, to which he mischievously retorted, 'Wrong answer. To walk with God you must go at walking pace.'"[7]

The words of Wang Mingdao touched me to the core. How can I talk about the Christian life as *walking* with God when I so often live it at a sprint? Of course we "run with perseverance the race marked out for us," but we may fail to run with "our eyes [fixed] on Jesus, the pioneer and perfecter of faith" (Heb 12:1-2). Jesus is inviting me to walk with him. Too often, I find myself running *for* him. There's a difference!

On another visit, Boyd-MacMillan asked Wang Mingdao about his twenty-year imprisonment for proclaiming Jesus in China. That cell became a place of unchosen unhurried time for Mingdao. There was nothing to do but to be in God's presence, which he discovered was actually *everything*. Boyd-MacMillan summarizes what he learned from Wang Mingdao:

> One of the keys to the faith of the suffering church: God does things slowly. He works with the heart. We are too quick. We have so much to do—so much in fact we never really commune with God as he intended when he created Eden, the perfect fellowship garden. For Wang Mingdao, persecution, or the cell in which he found himself, was the place where he returned to "walking pace," slowing down, stilling himself enough to commune properly with God.[8]

CLASSIC WISDOM FOR UNHURRIED LIVING

What counsel do I find in the Scriptures and Christian writings from centuries past for living a more unhurried life?

Psalm 46:10 offers us this unhurried invitation: "Be still, and know that I am God." Relax and remember who is in charge here.[9] Vincent de Paul, a seventeenth-century French priest dedicated to serving the poor, said, "[The one] who hurries delays the things of God." My usual pace of life reflects a different belief: "The one who hurries gets more done for God." Vincent claimed, however, that the person who hurries ahead in the things of God actually falls behind. But somehow we believe that hurry will hasten the things of God. What if Abraham hadn't rushed to help God keep his promise by having a child with Hagar (Gen 16)? Abraham's hurry caused serious delay of the things of God.

Proverbs 19:2 says, "Desire without knowledge is not good— how much more will hasty feet miss the way!" Here one of the costs of hurry is exposed. We feel the temptation some drivers feel: "I don't know where I am. What should I do? I know! I'll drive faster!" Hurrying like that puts us at risk of running past God's way for us. We somehow think that rushing about will put us on a fruitful path to God, but the opposite is usually true. Taking the unhurried way enables us to be attentive to God's presence and guidance. I want to learn to live at that pace of grace. No slower and definitely not any faster.

Author and pastor Wayne Muller tells the story of a South American tribe who would march for long periods and then abruptly sit and rest. When questioned about this pattern, they said "they needed the time of rest so that their souls could catch up with them."[10] Maybe being bored at times is a gift, an opportunity for those of us who go so fast we may be leaving our souls behind.

In his classic *Your God Is Too Small*, J. B. Phillips tells us that God is "never in a hurry."[11] Never in a hurry. How might a deeper awareness of God's gracious pacing transform our way of life and work? What would happen among us if we were to take on his unhurried manner? What might such a life look like? These are the questions I am bringing to these pages.

An Unhurried Journey with Jesus

I have come to appreciate the gifts of following an unhurried Savior. For example, I've found that a more unhurried inner pace decompresses my false sense of drivenness. I've also learned that "making things happen" isn't as helpful as learning to respond with courage to whatever God is doing. He makes things happen, and I would be wise to choose to work with him. My hurry is what often makes the yoke of life and ministry heavier than Jesus means it to be.

I find that when I am most hurried, I run past much that God is trying to show me, give me, lead me into. Hurry becomes my automatic-pilot modus operandi rather than a way to thrive in this life. I'm learning, as I watch Jesus' unhurried way, that keeping in step with him, living with him at a walking pace, is a way to sink into and enjoy the abundant life in him that he wants me to know.

So the question I would pose is this: If we are followers of an unhurried Savior, what should our pace of life look like? Since, for example, Jesus often stepped away from the needs of people to be alone with his Father in unhurried communion, might we, his followers, do well to learn to do the same? Being attentive to Jesus' life and learning from him can shape our vision of what the pace of grace will look like in our day-to-day lives. In some ways, living a Jesus-modeled, grace-paced life gets at the essence of spiritual leadership. I like to describe *spiritual leadership* as living a grace-paced life in the midst of a driven culture; living at a vital, life-giving, peaceful pace while remaining engaged and active in the kingdom work Jesus began here on this earth. I live not at the mercy of the culture's pace, but blessed by the mercy of my unhurried Savior.

An Overview of the Book

In this book, we will take a closer look at the idea that Jesus is an unhurried Savior. Chapter two looks at Jesus' unhurried way of developing apprentices. He sought to cultivate in his first followers an attentiveness to the Father that would enable them to influence people for Jesus far beyond their hopes or dreams. As I share my story of ministry leadership in a church setting, I want to offer insights you'll find helpful in the places of spiritual influence Jesus has entrusted to you as a parent, spiritual director, volunteer in your church or ministry leader. Next, chapter three looks at productivity and laziness and proposes that a more unhurried way of life is more productive than our often frantic and driven way. I also talk about *acedia,* a classic counterfeit to holy unhurry. Jesus' unhurried response to the temptations he faced in the wilderness will teach us how unhurry can protect us from impulsive actions that are less than life-giving (chapter four). A careful reading of Jesus' story of the good Samaritan will illustrate that being unhurried frees us to show compassion to the person right in front of us who is in need (chapter five). Chapter six explores Jesus' unhurried rhythm of prayer and ministry. He who often withdrew to lonely places to spend time in communion with the Father (Lk 5:16) encourages us to do the same: Jesus invites us to follow him in the rhythm of life he models for us.

In chapters seven through eleven, we will explore various facets of the unhurried way of life that Jesus invites us to share with him. Chapter seven talks about one of God's first gifts: during creation, he established the Sabbath, a day of rest. God later commanded his people to keep the Sabbath, a command Jesus fulfilled rather than abolished. In chapter eight, I share some of my experiences with suffering, an unwelcome reality in this fallen world that slows us down. In fact, nothing seems to slow our lives down quite as much as hardship or pain.

Chapter nine addresses Christian maturity, exposing the immaturity of our impulsivity and knee-jerk reactions. Maturity, however, does not happen overnight; it is, by nature, slow. Chapter ten offers some practical spiritual practices that can help us both cultivate a greater attentiveness to the presence of God in our lives and enjoy a simpler, richer walk with him. Finally, chapter eleven focuses on the ultimate in unhurried time—eternal life. How would our pace of life be affected if we fully realized that, as followers of Christ, we are living eternal life *now*? Since eternal life isn't just a dim future promise but a vital present reality, what could be different about how we live our moments and our days?

At the close of each chapter, in hopes of helping you enjoy the gift of an unhurried life, I will provide a few reflection questions that I call "Unhurried Time." In the spirit of our theme, I hope you'll take time to reflect on one of them before moving along to the next chapter. If you are reading this book in a group, you can also use these questions to reflect together. From experience, I can share that it is in experimenting and practicing that I've learned to welcome the grace of a less hurried heart, mind and manner.

Let me close with a prayer for us as we begin our journey toward unhurriedness: *Father, thank you for giving us, in your Son, an example of a grace-paced life. You know how much in bondage to the hurriedness of our culture we can feel. We want to live at the pace Jesus lived, but we are such slow learners. So please give us ears that hear you, hearts that are attentive to you and minds that are quiet before you so that we can learn from you. Living an unhurried way of life seems impossible, but, Almighty God, nothing is impossible for you. Amen.*

Unhurried Time

1. Think again about our cultural tendency to value a fast orientation and devalue a slow one. In what ways do you see this tendency in your own life? What voices, within or without, seek to keep you hurried? Why not take a few minutes to imagine in prayer how a more unhurried way might actually be a more fruitful one?

2. How do you respond to the idea of Jesus as relaxed? What is your initial reaction? Is it positive or negative? What changes would you like to see in your perspective here? Why not take a few moments to talk with Jesus about this?

3. In addition to some of the illustrations of Jesus' unhurried way that I've shared in this chapter, what others come to mind? What do these stories say about how you might be following Jesus in his way?

AN UNHURRIED APPRENTICE

When it comes to following Jesus and inviting others to join us on the journey, I hit a turning point in my life and ministry about twenty years ago. Up until that point, my ministry had been more about gathering a crowd than about cultivating a core of committed people and following Jesus together with them. My style of ministry was hurried and frantic. My goal was to fill the calendar with more events so I could fill the seats with more people. I would never have said it that bluntly, but it would have been hard for an objective observer to come to a different conclusion. I felt satisfied and important when the number of college students coming to our meetings was growing. I felt frustrated and worthless when that number decreased or even stayed the same. In conversations among our church staff at the time, we would say, "We count people because people count." I don't think that kind of math made anyone but us feel important, though.

At the beginning of that new season, when I was serving as a college pastor in a large church, I was introduced to the practice of spending extended time alone with God in silence, solitude and listening prayer. I had read many spiritual formation books affirming the value of such practices. I very much liked what they said, but I hadn't actually tried practicing those disciplines myself. I didn't quite know how to get there from where I found myself in my busy life and ministry. (Over the last twenty years, I have come across many who testify to having a similar experience.) This unhurried practice of extended time alone with God would, however, become essential to my growth as a follower of Jesus.

That day, the "extended time" was only seventy-five minutes. That was about all the leader of the retreat, Wayne Anderson, thought we seminarians could handle—and Wayne was probably right. A number of things happened in those minutes—and most of them in the last ten or fifteen. I spent the first hour feeling itchy and noisy inside. I found myself frustrated that God wasn't doing something or saying something to me. I expected, I suppose, some sort of burning bush, heavenly vision or inner voice—and I expected it in a hurry! What I experienced, however, was silence and solitude. To be fair, that was the advertised aim of the retreat day.

The main thing I remember about the time was that God brought to my mind a specific area of struggle—lust—that I needed to confess to my friend Chris, who was with me at the retreat. When that idea first crossed my mind during the time of solitude, I dismissed it. For one thing, I didn't want to be vulnerable in that way to anyone. For another, Chris was my college intern, and I didn't want him to see "Pastor Alan" in such a poor light. But I had told God at the beginning of the time that if there was anything I sensed him saying to me, I would write it down and take action on it.

So, on the hour-long drive home, I wrestled inside about admitting my struggle to Chris. We were at least halfway home when I began to tell him my story. It took a while. When I finished, he was silent. I began to think, *Oh no. What have I done? How will Chris ever trust me or respect me as his pastor?* Then, after a bit, Chris expressed appreciation for what I had shared and even began to talk about some places of need in his own life. That became a new place of growth in our journey as followers of Jesus. His grace began to touch these exposed places in our lives in vital and transformative ways that we hadn't experienced in our very busy schedules of ministry planning and activities.

A couple of days later, on Sunday afternoon, it was time for my weekly two-hour meeting with the college ministry team leaders. After talking through some details about a few upcoming events, I challenged these leaders to scatter around the church property and spend fifteen minutes alone and quiet with God, just listening to him. They were surprised by the assignment but, thankfully, willing.

This being a very new practice for me, I noticed as I wandered the church grounds that my mind didn't want to slow down. I was distracted by many things, and my mind kept wandering off— running off—in various directions. After a while, God seemed to bring the thought, *Slow down the pace.* I realized that my life and my work had been a kind of constant rush hour. I drove fast, walked fast, worked fast. Jesus was inviting me to slow down the pace of everything I did.

When I found myself slowing down inside, the Lord seemed to say, "Don't talk *trust* and live *worry.*" As a pastor, I often recommended truths that I was not practicing. Anxiety drove a lot of what I said and did. (Sometimes it still does.) And Jesus was inviting me to live with trust in him instead of worry.

As I walked back to my office to meet with the student leaders, God seemed to say, "Don't do homework tonight. Date your wife." I was behind on my seminary coursework, but my wife, Gem, had been gone for the whole weekend. I decided to listen to God, so later that evening, I shared with her more about my Friday encounter with Jesus. The seminary assignment eventually got done, but so much that was more important happened in this intimate conversation with my partner in life and ministry.

GOD SHOWS UP

After the group of leaders had reassembled, we shared with one another what we had experienced in our fifteen minutes alone and quiet with God. Brian, whom I had told about my Friday retreat, said that he had set aside some time on Saturday to be alone and quiet with the Lord. During that time an image came to his mind a couple of times, but he had disregarded it. Now, during this fifteen minutes of silence with the Lord on Sunday, the same image came up. It was the image of a balloon with a slow leak. As the balloon inevitably ran out of air, Brian was pumping it back up, over and over again. That picture helped him realize that he was living life in his own strength, pumping himself up for ministry, school and life. God was speaking to Brian about his need to find sustaining strength in God, rather than relying on his own strength that was so quickly depleted.

Other students talked about their fifteen minutes with God. Although I don't remember the specifics, I remember being overwhelmed by the power and reality of what each student experienced during the time. Fifteen minutes together planning a program or solving a problem would have been so much less significant than those fifteen unhurried minutes spent listening for God. And that listening would bear a great deal of fruit. It would change our understanding of the Christian life to a "following Jesus together" life.

The practices of solitude, silence and listening to God started to slow me down and enabled me to focus my attention more and more on coming to Jesus and following him rather than talking about Jesus and slaving away for him. In that context and over time, ministry became a matter of simply inviting students to join me in this journey. We were learning to follow Jesus together. The focus was less and less on our activities *for* him and more on our attentiveness *to* him, on walking *with* him, and on working *with* him. We were learning together how to follow him—and it was one of the hardest years of my life and ministry. In many ways, my previous focus on planning more events and giving more talks was easier. Staying busy seemed easier than becoming unhurried, at least at the time. And it was a lot less messy.

One of the transitions we made in our college ministry that year was that my wife, Gem, and I began to focus our attention on a small group of student leaders. About a dozen of them—young men and women who, like me, had been very hurried in planning all of the events and meetings and trips for our college ministry—joined us in seeking Christ together in the context of our leadership gatherings. Often we would take thirty minutes of a two-hour meeting to go our separate ways and simply be alone with God. Depending on where we were meeting, we would walk the church property or around our neighborhood. We'd either listen to what God was saying to us personally through a passage of Scripture or just wait on God together in a heart posture of attentive listening. I wanted to assume that the students could do this on their own time, but we discovered that our way of life and ministry up until then made that unlikely. We needed to learn together how to live this "Come to me, come follow me" way of life.

When we began to focus on Christ like this during our leadership gatherings, when we listened for what God had to say to us and prayed for the larger community of students we served, we realized that being unhurried before God was a messy proposition. Personal struggles surfaced. Conflicts arose. It may sound strange, but we weren't accustomed to being that involved in one another's lives. We were used to staying busy with the work, but that year it wasn't uncommon for us to spend a large portion of these weekly meetings addressing those personal struggles and interpersonal issues. Sometimes two or three smaller meetings would be occurring as small groups of students hashed out their hurts and sins. Sometimes a few students would gather around to pray for another who had confessed a particular struggle that had been, until then, hidden by the busyness of doing ministry.

At the end of that year, Gem and I took a group of students across the country to Urbana, InterVarsity Christian Fellowship's triennial missions conference. In one of the sessions, we were given five or ten minutes to be silent and listen for God together. There were about eighteen thousand of us in that assembly hall. During those few minutes, God seemed to be giving both my wife and me a vision, which was odd, because we didn't expect God to do things like that anymore! Later that day, Gem shared that she had seen an image of us in a room full of leaders, first her alone with women and me alone with men, then both of us together with the whole group. We were simply sharing our lives. We were telling our stories. In my vision, I had seen what looked like a large map, a grid, with all of the squares grayed out except the bottom left one. It looked like a fully developed map with streets, rivers and other features. I knew inside that it was an image of a future ministry of expanded influence.

Realize that Gem and I were in our late twenties at that time. We didn't yet have much life experience to share with others. Over time, though, we've come to realize that these visions were an invitation to develop followers of Jesus by becoming his followers ourselves and then inviting others to join us in the journey. Our visions invited us to step off the ministry hamster wheel we had made for ourselves and instead take on the easy and well-fitting yoke of Jesus for our lives and our ministry—and then to help others do the same. That choice has made all the difference. As a result of that choice, we began to think differently—and perhaps less hurriedly—about our focus in ministry.

The Problem of the Crowd

Elton Trueblood, an influential spiritual writer and philosopher of the mid-1900s whose writings I have valued, once wrote a chapter titled "The Problem of the Crowd." In it he wisely noted:

> Jesus refused to depend upon crowds for the obvious reason
> that He knew them to be undependable. There is nothing in
> all this to suggest any snobbishness or any failure to appre-
> ciate the importance of each single individual among the five
> thousand. Instead, the meaning is the simple one that mere
> mass movements do not usually make any permanent im-
> pression. The permanent impression, if it comes, has to come
> in some other way. Christ's reason for turning away from the
> crowds was not any lack of love for persons, but an intense
> concern for a cause. We have good evidence that Christ loved
> the people in the crowds and had deep sympathy for them.
> This is suggested by the sentence, "When he saw the crowds,
> he had compassion for them, because they were harassed and
> helpless, like sheep without a shepherd." He was so touched
> by their pain and confusion that it must have been difficult to
> turn from them, again and again, in order to pray alone or to
> instruct the inner group.[1]

I have a confession to make: unlike Jesus, I'm tempted to appeal
to the crowd. (You don't need to have a paid ministry role to feel
that temptation.) I like hearing lots of people say nice things about
me. I want the crowd to like me. And the apparent advantage of
appealing to the crowd is that I can gain what feels like quick influence. But none of this is about helping people follow Jesus. It's
about serving my self-interest and pursuing my personal ambition
to be seen as an impressive person.

On the other hand, like Jesus, I long to help those in the crowd
realize that they don't always know what they want or need. We're
all tempted to come to Jesus for what we want from him, rather
than coming to him for mentoring, training and teaching about
what he wants our lives to look like. This kind of apprentice devel-

opment takes time: it involves long-term transformation. I know that my own growth in following Jesus more closely hasn't happened quickly, and a focus on helping others follow Jesus more closely doesn't look very impressive in the short-term. Even Jesus didn't seem to have much to show for his efforts after three years. But in Jesus' case, his influence and impact has borne kingdom fruit for centuries beyond his human lifetime.

Think of ministry events or gatherings in your life. You may be a participant or you may be a leader. When people gather, we hope that everyone coming wants help in learning how to grow in following Jesus. But is this why everyone comes? And if it isn't, why do I think they'll change their minds about what they want once they do come? It makes little sense to attract people on the basis of their own self-interest and then expect them to embrace an invitation to self-denial. Furthermore, if my aim is to gather and keep a crowd, I will avoid any risk of communicating the difficult yet life-giving message of self-denial, even if it is the path to a richer life than I could ever find on my own.

When I think about the crowds that followed Jesus, I realize that they came to Jesus not to listen to his teaching or to know him better. They came for what they wanted from him. They didn't come interested in what he wanted for them, and this reality sparked conflict between Jesus and the crowds. Crowds tend to be self-interested. Crowds come and go. Crowds are fickle and unpredictable. What collects a crowd one day may well disperse it the next. Crowds that love us today may hate us tomorrow. Yet we can quickly gather a crowd when we attract them on the basis of what they want—or at least what they *think* they want.

Well aware of that aspect of human nature, Jesus, through careful prayer, selected an inner circle of twelve from among the many who were coming to him early on so that they would be with him all the time. They would join him in a three-year journey that

would transform their lives. They gazed upon God-in-the-flesh.
Don't we want to be part of ministries today that help focus people's attention on Jesus himself?

THE FICKLE CROWD

Now let's consider how Jesus' evaluation of the crowds and his apparent attempt to often avoid them differs from our common attempt to gather and even cater to the crowd whenever possible. Jesus attracted crowds very early in his ministry, and soon he seemed to try to avoid them. It wasn't that he didn't care for the individuals who comprised those multitudes, but they wanted something from Jesus that he didn't want to focus his attention on. They wanted him to be a meal ticket or a magician—anything but Savior, Lord and God! The crowds were not following him for transformation, but for benefits. Their motivation was far more outward than inward. And their excitement about Jesus would only last as long as he gave them what they wanted.

If Jesus had wanted to, he could have gathered tens of thousands of people around him with little effort. No one was a more engaging speaker. No one else had the miraculous abilities that Jesus had. But he did not appear interested in gathering a crowd. He focused instead on developing a small circle of devoted apprentices.

Despite Jesus' example, I find it a continual temptation to do things that will get a lot of people excited about what I'm doing—and get them excited now! Even though I am well aware of the fickle nature of a crowd, it's far harder to persevere in the long-term work of developing a few followers who will grow in their allegiance to Jesus.

A brief survey of Jesus' interaction with crowds reveals how unpredictable and unreliable they are. When Jesus began his ministry, for instance, the crowds were impressed by his spiritual power and gracious words (Lk 4:14-15). But when Jesus challenged their agenda, members of that same crowd reacted and were ready to throw him off a cliff (Lk 4:24-30). News of his amazing wisdom in teaching and his power in healing continued to draw crowds (Lk 5:15). At about that same time, Luke points out, Jesus often withdrew to lonely (uncrowded?) places to pray (Lk 5:16). Another time, a crowd welcomed Jesus into their town, almost crushing him in an attempt to get close to him (Lk 8:40-42). But when Jesus said that the daughter of a synagogue leader he had come to heal wasn't dead but just sleeping, the crowd ridiculed and mocked him (Lk 8:53). It doesn't take much to turn a sympathetic crowd into a scorning crowd.

Later, Jesus warned the crowd about the wickedness of the present generation (Lk 11:29). Another time, he said to the crowds, "If anyone comes to me and does not hate father and mother, wife and children, brothers and sisters—yes, even their own life—such a person cannot be my disciple. And whoever does not carry their cross and follow me cannot be my disciple" (Lk 14:26-27). Jesus continued to extend an invitation to the crowds to follow him and not just seek from him what they wanted. During his travels, still accompanied by a crowd, a blind man cried out for Jesus to have mercy on him. The crowd rebuked him, something Jesus wouldn't do (Lk 18:35-40). The crowd traveled with Jesus, but they weren't *following* him. And of course the crowd convinced Pilate not to release Jesus, but demanded that he be crucified instead (Lk 23:18-24). The crowd that praised Jesus with "Hosanna!" one day was later shouting, "Crucify him!"

So is the way we engage in ministry, whether as pastors, volunteer leaders or other spiritual servants, more oriented toward attracting a crowd or making apprentices of Jesus? One way we can determine that is to consider the standards we use to measure "success." Do our conversations about ministry revolve around growing numbers of participants, successful programs or other easily measured outcomes? Or do we tell stories about particular people who are responding to Jesus, stories of seeds of gospel truth sown in people's hearts that will grow into the fruit of Christlikeness?

Crowds also validate our work in a hurry. We want to make a difference, but we want to make a difference in a way that can be measured right away. Programs attended by crowds of people are "successful" and serve as a kind of currency that proves the worth of our church or ministry group. We want to see growth. Who doesn't? But in our North American context, quantitative growth of just about *any* kind is the primary ruler used to measure and validate a ministry. More people, more buildings, more dollars, more programs—these are considered evidence of divine blessing. Those servants who can't do any bragging about quantitative progress are assumed to be failing at doing God's work well. Since it's hard to patiently work with people long enough that they become deeply rooted followers of Jesus, we too often settle for helping them learn more information rather than focusing on the long, hard work of equipping them to follow Jesus. Such "growth" is easier to quantify, and the results of our efforts are more quickly seen. But righteousness involves far more than just knowing what's right: righteousness means living well. And that takes time to learn.

Our ministries tend to use crowd-building strategies to grow because, if we have great speaking or sizzling programs, a crowd soon gathers. They did during Jesus' life and ministry, and he had great compassion for the members of the crowd. Jesus saw them as sheep without a shepherd, and he longed to shepherd them well. Yet the crowd wasn't coming to him on his terms, but on theirs. They wanted what they wanted from this miracle worker. Jesus, however, wanted to invest God's truth and love in people who would trust him, follow him, be shepherded by him and be apprenticed to him.

Apprenticeship and Spiritual Leadership

What kind of spiritual leadership helps to develop men and women who are growing in their apprenticeship to Jesus? What does it look like? How does it work? How can we be part of such a movement? The apostle Paul told potential followers to "follow my example, as I follow the example of Christ" (1 Cor 11:1), but to what degree would I feel confident inviting people to live their lives the way I live mine? Also, is my vision of spiritual leadership limited to the words I speak, or am I coming to more and more embody the way of life I proclaim? What am I doing to let my life be shaped by God and his priorities for me rather than misshaped by cultural pressures?

Furthermore, if I understand leadership to be, in large part, influence, then spiritual leadership is spiritual influence. We must consider: what kind of influence is my life having on the people God has placed around me and on how they live their lives? Is my life different enough to provoke or inspire others to change their way of life? Spiritual leadership—spiritual modeling—isn't a prideful "Look at me!" invitation. It is instead a "Look to Christ as I am learning to do" invitation. What aspect of the presence of Christ being formed in me, if any, is tantalizing and able to draw others to follow my example? At the same time, in what negative ways has my life influenced others? What spiritually unhealthy, distracted or willful ways have I modeled?

Do I believe that the very presence of Christ being formed in me and filling me is the greatest resource I have as I ask the Lord to use me to influence others to become his followers? If so, what kind of attention am I giving to my own following of him? When it comes to having a positive spiritual influence, am I living as a person of integrity? Is who I appear to be on the outside in harmony with who I am on the inside? If not, my life will lack integrity. I want to be as rich in soul as I try to appear to others. Besides, I might have more influence on fellow believers if I am honest about my struggles instead of pretending that I have none!

So, when it comes to being unhurried enough to develop a community of people who will walk and work with Jesus, what can we learn from the most often-quoted passage on making disciples?

Two Great Commissions

Paul Jensen, founder of The Leadership Institute and my colleague, has written on what he calls the dual commission of Matthew 28. That passage is, of course, where we hear Jesus charge his followers to *go and make disciples of all nations.* Jensen urges us to see this commission in context. He wants to widen our view of what Jesus commanded to include verses 16-20 (most treatments of the Great Commission begin with verse 18):

> Then the eleven disciples went to Galilee, to the mountain where Jesus had told them to go. When they saw him, they worshiped him; but some doubted. Then Jesus came to them and said, "All authority in heaven and on earth has been given to me. Therefore go and make disciples of all nations, baptizing them in the name of the Father and of the Son and of the Holy Spirit, and teaching them to obey everything I have commanded you. And surely I am with you always, to the very end of the age."

Jensen suggests that, if we see Jesus' commission to us in this broader biblical context, we will make this "obvious observation":

> There are two commissions here, an inner and outer one. First Jesus directed his disciples to the mountain—there to meet him, see him, worship him, and experience his unconditional love, especially in their doubt (or perhaps hesitation). Second, in the context of their obedience to the inner commission, he gave them the outer commission to make disciples of all nations.[2]

When it comes to fulfilling what we've often called the Great

Commission, have we done so with a rich sense of Jesus' presence with us, worshiping his majesty in humility and acknowledging our honest doubts or hesitations as we see him there on the mountain where he delivered the charge? Do we remember that, rather than helping people follow Jesus in whatever way seems best to us, we are to act under his authority and remain in him as we do so? (To be honest, I'm afraid that I have, in the past, tried to carry out this commission of Jesus without much communion with him. It has been much activity without much abiding.)

Then, as we reflect on the charge in particular, at what point does our tendency to hurry interfere? Many have presumed that the main point of Jesus' command is *go*. But the structure of the original language carries more the sense of "*As you go*, make disciples of all nations." The main charge is the making of disciples, the invitation to work with people from every nation who will choose to follow Jesus. But what will this look like?

First, it will involve baptizing them in the name of the Father and of the Son and of the Holy Spirit, what Dallas Willard paraphrases as "surrounding them, immersing them in the reality of the Trinitarian community."[3] I spent my earliest Christian years in Baptist-flavored churches, and we tended to reduce this aspect of making disciples to an argument about how wet new Christians were supposed to get. We also condensed making disciples into a single event that, meaningful as it was, was soon left behind as we moved new believers on to the next things. But a less hurried approach might be to help new followers focus on how to be more immersed in the presence of Jesus, to share this way of life together as a primary focus.

After speaking about baptism, Jesus then called us to "[teach] them to obey everything I have commanded you." Sometimes it has seemed that I was only intentional about teaching potential or new believers *what* to obey without teaching them much about *how* to obey. Perhaps I didn't know how to obey Jesus well myself. It doesn't take long to teach *what*. Teaching *how* requires a more unhurried, personalized approach, and it is far more challenging. Yet such a one-on-one and small-group approach is how apprentices learn to do well what they are being trained to do. This approach is also more fruitful: I teach those who now call themselves Christ-followers how *good* it is to obey—how life-giving and fruitful—and I help them realize how much, in the new heart God created within them, they really *want* to obey.

Jesus' commission closes with these words: "And surely I am with you always, to the very end of the age." How well do we remember this truth? Do we slow down enough in our desire to carry out what Jesus calls us to do to remember that he is with us as we do it? We are never alone, we are never abandoned and we are never a lone ranger in anything we do in service to God's kingdom.

The Great Commission takes us to the end of Jesus' earthly ministry and his invitation to "make disciples." But what about the beginning of his ministry?

ISAIAH 61: OAKS OF RIGHTEOUSNESS

Early in his ministry, Jesus visited the synagogue in Nazareth, his hometown. There, he stood up and read from the Isaiah scroll:

> The Spirit of the Lord is on me,
>   because he has anointed me
>   to proclaim good news to the poor.
> He has sent me to proclaim freedom for the prisoners
>   and recovery of sight for the blind,
>   to set the oppressed free,
>   to proclaim the year of the Lord's favor. (Lk 4:18-19)

Then Jesus said, "Today this scripture is fulfilled in your hearing" (verse 21). In other words, Jesus was saying, "This is what I've come to do. This is what I'm about." He chose not to continue reading on in the scroll where Isaiah next said "and to proclaim . . . the day of vengeance of our God" (Is 61:2). If Jesus had continued reading that passage, one that was very familiar to his listeners, he would have come to these lines:

They will be called oaks of righteousness,
a planting of the LORD
for the display of his splendor. (Is 61:3)

This is, to me, an apprenticeship metaphor. Isaiah was not describing a situation where people in need merely find their need met in the Messiah. The prophet was describing a situation where the needy, broken, enslaved and despairing become oaks of righteousness.

Isaiah envisioned a kingdom in which those people in need of grace become, over time, solidly rooted in God's grace, enough so as to be able to extend his grace to others. He envisioned a kingdom where we would experience favor, comfort, blessing, honor, new perspectives and deepening roots that enable us to do the rebuilding, restoring, renewing work in places, structures and persons who have long been ruined (Is 61:4). These characteristics of oaks of righteousness are the fruit of apprenticeship. Further, we, as these oaks of righteousness planted by the Lord, put his splendor on display, a display quite different from human excitement, enthusiasm and thrills. *Splendor* is quieter, stronger, less hurried and more deeply rooted.

Oaks take a long time to grow. A newly planted acorn can take between two and three decades to provide significant shade, and these slow-growing oaks can live more than two hundred years. One reason for their longevity is the taproot they send deep into the earth that makes them very drought-resistant. Oaks are indeed solid, stable, reliable, majestic trees—but it takes them a while to get there. Do we take that same long view of growing in Christ ourselves and helping others do the same? If so, what can we do to help others become attentive and teachable apprentices to him so that one day they will shine with his splendor and flourish in the fruit of his Spirit? Whatever it is that we do, I believe it will require a less hurried, longer perspective approach than we have commonly taken.

When we first begin to follow Jesus, we have not yet become oaks of righteousness. We are more like the poor, brokenhearted and captive people Isaiah describes. But Jesus intends to transform us dramatically. He wants us to come to reflect the beauty, goodness and rootedness of an oak tree. He's planted us. He will tend us. He will do what it takes to deepen and strengthen our roots in him. That's a pretty dramatic transformation. How much time and effort does this kind of change take? In my experience, it doesn't happen in a hurry.

CONCLUSION

When we reach the end of this earthly journey, what will we look back on with joy and gratitude? What will we look back on with sadness and even regret? I don't think I'll find my deepest joy in the number of people who liked something I said or did. I'm coming to believe that my greatest joy will be being part of an extended community of men and women with whom I've shared a journey with Jesus, living out his life in our families, our neighborhoods, our workplaces and schools, and the church communities where God has planted us. I will celebrate their rootedness, their fruitfulness and their deep, Christlike influence on the lives of others with all my heart.

Becoming an apprentice of Jesus is a lifelong journey. He will use every day of my life to transform me, inside and out, using whatever life-giving ways he wants to use. And our efforts to help others become followers of Jesus take time as well. Helping others learn to walk with Jesus and not stop at just believing things about him requires intentionality and focused effort. We never *find* time to do this patient work. We must *make* time. Unhurried time.

UNHURRIED TIME

1. When you think about ministries you lead or are part of, how much of your assigned work is meant to draw and maintain a crowd? How much intentional effort do you pour into growing individuals whose allegiance to Jesus is deepening, enabling him to transform their character and lives? What aspects of your work will produce lasting fruit?

2. In what ways do you see busyness in your life—even in your Christian life or ministry life—as more of a hindrance to your following Jesus than a help?

3. What opportunities to simplify your life might Jesus be inviting you to consider so that you can walk more closely with him and share the riches of that journey with other like-minded Christ-followers?

PRODUCTIVITY

Unhurried Isn't Lazy

When a young child is about to put her hand on a hot stove, we don't unhurriedly stroll over to see what might happen. We jump into action to protect the child from harm. In this situation, hurry is holy.

Emergencies call for a rapid response. I think of biblical stories that illustrate this idea. When God is about to rain down judgment on Sodom and Gomorrah, Lot urges his sons-in-law, "Hurry and get out of this place" (Gen 19:14). Joseph, during a great famine, urges his brothers to hurry home to their father and bring him back to Egypt, where they can find food (Gen 45:9). Some of Pharaoh's officials who begin to believe in the word Moses is speaking on God's behalf hurry to take their slaves and livestock inside before the plague of hail falls (Ex 9:20). Later, the Egyptians urge the Israelites to leave right away before the plagues kill the entire nation (Ex 12:33). Moses urges Aaron to hurry and make an atonement offering to God in response to the consequences of Korah's rebellion against Moses and his leadership (Num 16:46).

Hurry makes sense in an emergency, and emergencies happen. People get injured or sick and need to be hurried to the hospital.

Urgent issues arise that require immediate attention and quick action. The problem is when we find ourselves living with a *constant* sense of urgency; we get stuck there. *Every* situation feels like an emergency, whether it is or not. Our bodies weren't meant to live at such a constant level of alertness, and our souls don't function well in such a mode. But neither are we meant to waste our days.

WHEN UNHURRY IS UNHOLY

There is, of course, an unhurry that is unholy. While there is the waiting to which God invites us, there is another kind of waiting that is our resistance to God's invitation. Delay in responding to clear counsel from God is not the kind of unhurry I'm recommending. Such unhurry is a failure to appreciate that *today*—not tomorrow—is the day of salvation. Being unhurried does not at all mean being unresponsive to divine nudges. Being unhurried enables us to notice those nudges and to respond.

When I talk about an unhurried life, I am not talking about a *lazy* life. Proverbs offers many words of warning to the lazy, these among them:

> Go to the ant, you sluggard;
> consider its ways and be wise!
> It has no commander,
> no overseer or ruler,
> yet it stores its provisions in summer
> and gathers its food at harvest.
> How long will you lie there, you sluggard?
> When will you get up from your sleep?
> A little sleep, a little slumber,
> a little folding of the hands to rest—
> and poverty will come on you like a thief
> and scarcity like an armed man. (Prov 6:6-11)

A sluggard is guilty of underwork whereas the workaholic is guilty of overwork. Where are we to fall on this spectrum? Solomon urges us to learn a lesson about fruitful labor from one of our smallest neighbors—the ant. Without any coaching, the ant stores food for itself when there is plenty so that it will have what it needs in times of want. The ant does not procrastinate and put off until tomorrow—or later today or an hour from now—what can be done well now. And what is done now, in the present moment, can be done with an unhurried heart.

Holy leisure and unholy idleness are polar opposites. This sort of idleness isn't life-giving. It isn't good. It isn't God's way. But I am recommending that we consider stepping off the treadmill or out of the fast lane long enough to relax and linger in God's presence, to walk with him at his pace. This *isn't* being lazy. Jesus himself knew how to get out of the fray so he could linger with the Father. Remember our one-word description of Jesus? *Relaxed*—and relaxed is not the same as sleepy. Relaxed can be very attentive and engaged. A sprinter standing in the starting blocks is both ready and relaxed at the same time. Jesus modeled for us not only how to withdraw and linger in God's presence, but also how to relax in it.

Despite this divine precedent and example, we're often tempted to think that unhurry *equals* laziness. For example, Gerald May suggests that our efficiency-orientation makes unhurried times for rest feel selfish, irresponsible and lazy: "We know we need rest, but we can no longer see the value of rest as an end in itself; it is only worthwhile if it helps us recharge our batteries."[1] Unhurry and laziness are not equivalents. Jesus was unhurried, but he was not lazy. He was engaged, hardworking, purposeful and conscientious.

Brenda Ueland helps us distinguish between healthy unhurry and empty idleness:

If your idleness is a complete slump, that is, indecision, fretting, worry, or due to over-feeding and physical mugginess, that is bad, terrible and utterly sterile. Or if it is that idleness which so many people substitute for creative idleness, such as gently feeding into their minds all sorts of printed bilge like detective stories and newspapers, that is too bad and utterly uncreative.[2]

Unholy unhurry is sterile, empty and lifeless rather than fruitful, significant and life-giving.

ACEDIA: UNHOLY UNHURRY

Another form of unholy unhurry that many of us have heard little about is *acedia*. Derived from the Greek *a* (for "not") and *keedos* (meaning "to care"), acedia is ultimately a failure of love. It's a place of apathy toward life and a kind of spiritual boredom; it's that umpteenth lap somewhere between the enthusiasm of the starting line and the celebration of the finish line. Whether midday, midlife, halftime or halfway through a big project, we're tempted to give in, give up or distract ourselves.

Acedia tempts us to abandon the life we have for some imagined better option somewhere else—as in "anywhere but here"! Acedia can also be the temptation to live our lives in imagined fantasies of what *might be* rather than living in the gift of what *is*. Though it may seem unhurried from a certain perspective, acedia is rooted in a restless, distracted and, yes, hurried heart.

In *Acedia and Me*, Kathleen Norris suggests the likelihood "that much of the restless boredom, frantic escapism, commitment phobia, and enervating despair that plague us today is the ancient demon of acedia in modern dress."[3] Sound familiar?

Evagrius Ponticus, a fourth-century monk who offered key insights into acedia, described those afflicted as feeling that the "sun

hardly moves and that the day is fifty hours long; the monk constantly looks out the window, walks around outside, peers at the
sun to figure out how long until dinner time; there arises a dislike
for the place, for the monastic life, for work; the monk thinks that
love has fled from among the brothers and that there is no one to
provide any encouragement."[4]

Acedia tempts us to camp in lethargic fantasy or rush along to
some imagined "grass is greener" meadow. Anything but here and
now. It's a kind of soul-weariness in the midst of our journey, a loss
of holy desire that would energize the practices by which we make
open space and unhurried time in our life so we notice the real
presence of God. He is always with you and me, yet we don't always
remain aware of this most basic of spiritual facts. We behave too
often as though God either isn't present or is so distant that his
presence is irrelevant.

A spiritual malaise, acedia causes us to find spiritual disciplines
boring and not worth our time. It is a loss of a more eternal perspective: we forget that we are living eternal life now. Living each
moment in the light of eternity enables us to remain unhurried and
engaged in the work God has for us in the present moment. We
human beings are easily tempted to escape our responsibilities
and, for that matter, to suppress any responsiveness to God. Our "I
don't feel like it" is an unholy indifference.

Since acedia is a failure to appreciate the gifts of the present
moment or the present season, the classic remedy for acedia has
always been to abide in the good relationships and to engage in the
good work before us. We counter acedia's enticement to seek some
unknown better that lies anywhere but here with an intentional
and positive focus on the present. Benedictine professor Columba
Stewart says that "Benedict prescribes service of one another,
mutual obedience, work, spiritual guidance and annual renewal in
Lent as ways to keep monastic life grounded in the freshness of

each moment."[5] These are ways of living and savoring the life we've been given rather than dreaming about or searching for a life we imagine as better than this one.

So, at its simplest, the opposite of acedia is love—devotion to Christ that produces active, sincere, engaged concern for others. If we let our thoughts wander, the sharpness of our holy concern will be dulled by lust, envy, greed or other unholy, lazy inward impulses.

These days, acedia sometimes sneaks up behind me, often in the middle of my day, and whispers something like, "Haven't you done enough work on that presentation or that retreat? You'd be fresher tomorrow. Why don't you check a few of your favorite websites? See what's happening on Facebook and Twitter. See if anyone is visiting your blog. Take a little break with one of your favorite video games." When I follow the unholy spiritual counsel acedia proposes, I end up in fruitless, joyless, lifeless places. I cease to engage in the hard, good work God prepared well in advance for this very day.

In contrast to the fruitlessness of acedia's counsel, I find the fruitfulness of God's Spirit a life-giving antidote. Just before Paul lists the fruit of the Spirit in Galatians 5, he offers a list of what our flesh—that element of us that has been formed in resistance and disconnection from the Spirit—promotes apart from the Spirit.

Love: Apart from the Spirit, I become disengaged and selfish, hating and being hated, uninvolved and uncaring. What do I really care about? Who really matters to me? Caring doesn't hurry.

Joy: Apart from the Spirit, I become depressed, or I seek thrills instead of holy delight. I become slothful, even exhausted. I become narrowed in my perspective and cynical. Joy withers in my hurry to amuse myself. What will instead energize me and give me holy pleasure?

Peace: Apart from the Spirit, I become worried and anxious, hurried and stressed, frazzled and frayed. Where and when do I feel a deep sense of well-being and rest? Peace is a fruit of unhurriedness.

Patience: Apart from the Spirit, I easily lose my temper. In no time I become intolerant and irritated. I find that every little issue in the lives of others can provoke me. Patience is the opposite of hurry.

Kindness: Apart from the Spirit, I fail to offer even simple courtesy to others. I become mean, harsh and calloused. True kindness takes unhurried time.

Goodness: Apart from the Spirit, my goodness becomes self-righteousness. I find myself titillated by innuendo, mired in double-mindedness, unwholesome and unhealthy in my choices. Goodness is a fruit of unhurried communion with God, the only One who is good.

Faithfulness: Apart from the Spirit, I can become flaky, burned out and unreliable. Faithfulness is evident in unhurried commitment, a long obedience in the same direction.

Gentleness: Apart from the Spirit, I become sharp and harsh with others, demanding and unsympathetic. Gentleness isn't in a harsh hurry.

Self-Control: Apart from the Spirit, I spin out of control. I become enslaved to pleasure, power and empty amusement. Self-control resists the rush to get what I crave.

The genuine productivity of the Spirit is the fruit of an unhurried orientation to God and to people. My life with God and my relationships with people need more unhurried time in order to be rooted in him and therefore fruitful. I see this truth in Nicodemus's comment to Jesus: "No one could perform the [miraculous] signs you are doing if God were not with him" (Jn 3:2). Nicodemus recognized in the works of Jesus that God's favor was with him. In fact, Nicodemus was seeing in Jesus both the works of the Father and the fruit of God's Spirit.

Do you find yourself mired in the unholy unhurry of acedia? If you're not sure, stop. Listen. Ask yourself, *What is the good in this present moment that I can notice, acknowledge, enjoy and share with a trusted friend? What good work lies right here before me, disguised initially as something boring?* Listen. Then step into that good work. Walk with God in it.

How Productive Is Overwork Really?

Speaking of life in the marketplace, Carl Honoré, in his book *In Praise of Slowness,* makes this observation:

> Of course, speed has a role in the workplace. A deadline can focus the mind and spur us on to perform remarkable feats. The trouble is that many of us are permanently stuck in deadline mode, leaving little time to ease off and recharge. The things that need slowness—strategic planning, creative thought, building relationships—get lost in the mad dash to keep up, or even just to look busy.[6]

An unhurried orientation to life does not prevent us from doing work quickly and well. Sitting around, failing to engage in the good work God has entrusted to us is not good. We know this. There is something satisfying when all of our cylinders are engaged and we are moving along at a good clip. When we know what God is inviting us to and engage it with whole hearts and all our energy, there is a pleasure and joy we find in no other way. The problem comes when our accelerator is stuck and we no longer know the way to fill needs that can only be met in slowness.

A primary resistance to a less hurried way of life—a resistance I find in myself and in others—is the belief that "I won't be as productive" or that "I will fail to seize the opportunities God sets before me." I have come to believe, though, that this sort of obsession with work results, ironically, in a reduction of true fruitfulness. We sometimes hear it said, "Less is more." Sometimes, though, more is also less.

This question of overwork reminds me of what Jesus said about his own work. Responding to complaints by the Jewish leaders that he was healing people—doing work—on the Sabbath, Jesus explained, "My Father is always at his work to this very day, and I too am working. . . . Very truly I tell you, the Son can do nothing by himself; he can do only what he sees his Father doing, because whatever the Father does the Son also does" (Jn 5:17, 19).

Jesus saw himself as an apprentice to the Father in his work. He was not working on his own. Whatever he did was something he had seen his Father working at. I fear, therefore, that my own overwork is a failure of discernment. Am I following Jesus in my own way of working? Is all the work I'm doing in keeping with what the Father is doing and how he is doing it? Do I know what the Father is doing in the lives of people around me who are affected by my work? Am I working in concert with the Father or, perhaps unaware, in conflict with him? Might I find myself *overdoing* something God may later have to *undo*?

Hearing that Jesus can do nothing by himself, but only what he sees his Father doing, makes me think of Jesus' own words to me: "Apart from me you can do nothing" (Jn 15:5). I long to do all the good work God has for me, like the work he is doing in me, through me and around me. Am I, however, discerning what that is? I have noticed, after all, that apart from him I can still be very busy, just not very fruitful. My overwork is just another example of accelerating even though I'm lost.

Something else I notice about Jesus' work may seem so obvious as to need no further comment: his work directly affected people. He taught them. He healed them. He released them from their captivity. Good work helps others. So much of my overwork is many stages removed from directly blessing people. It's often just busywork. And busywork isn't usually productive work. When that's the case, my overwork feels like a whole lot of prospecting to try to gather a little gold dust.

With our modern way of working accelerated by the power of technology, just how fruitful are we? In her book *Sloth*, Wendy Wasserstein asks, "Are these hyperscheduled, overactive individuals really creating anything new? Are they guilty of passion in any way? Do they have a new vision for their government? For their community? Or for themselves?" It seems "their purpose is to keep themselves so busy, so entrenched in their active lives, that their spirit reaches a permanent state of lethargiosis."[7] Overwork can end up like progress made on a treadmill. Furthermore, there can be an ironic laziness about such work. The sheer quantity may be impressive, but quantity does not require as much effort from us as work that results in creativity, vitality or joy. In that sense, overwork can be lazy work.

In contrast, I remember a visit to a small village in the western mountains of the Dominican Republic. A friend and I enjoyed the hospitality of a young family living very simply in a nearby home in Manabao. The house was built on a simple cement slab, painted dark green and kept very clean. The walls were rough-cut local lumber, the ceiling was a single layer of corrugated sheet metal, and the furnishings were simple and functional. The whole house for this extended family of at least seven was smaller than many North American master bedrooms. The wife and homemaker, Ellie, prepared us a delicious lunch of rice, beans and a little bit of chicken (which had been running around the village earlier that day) cooked over an open, smoky fire.

My friend and translator, Samuel, asked Julio, Ellie's husband, whether he would like to move into the city with all of the conveniences and resources there. Julio's answer was something like this: "I like the peace and quiet of this area. My family has everything we need. I like raising my children here and spending time with them. I notice that rich people buy land out here and build big houses so they can come and rest on the weekends. I get to live out here every day. I wouldn't trade places with them."

I don't want to glamorize or idealize what, for some, is a very challenging existence. The poor often need help just to sustain their lives. They often do not have ready access to medical help. A friend of mine who lives and works among the urban poor of Buenos Aires, Argentina, notices a great sense of hurry connected to sheer survival there. Of course the poor do not share a single, simple story. I found that Julio and Ellie were living a fruitful life, doing fruitful work, even if it was simple and unimpressive by certain standards. They were peaceful and joyful. As we asked and they answered our questions, Julio had his arm around Ellie, and there was an unmistakable richness that too many North Americans lack—the richness of time and space to enjoy life, enjoy people, even enjoy God.

That conversation highlights for me a certain poverty in my hurried way as one who is wealthy in comparison with so much of the world. I see this insight brought into focus in a word Jesus spoke to a wealthy person in the crowd: "Watch out! Be on your guard against all kinds of greed; life does not consist in an abundance of possessions" (Lk 12:15). A good life, a rich life, an abundant life *does not* consist in having more material goods. But I live in a culture that is based on the assumption that this is *exactly* how our lives get better. And because this is a deep cultural assumption, I rarely question it, even though it drives me to work harder to make more money to acquire more goods to have what I assume is a better life. The drive to possess is an engine for hurry.

I have come to find that, like many North Americans, I may be wealthy compared to the rest of the world, but I am at the same time quite poor. In the words of author Robert Banks, "While American society is rich in goods, it is extremely time-poor. Many societies in the two-thirds world, by contrast, are poor in material possessions, by our standards, but they are rich in time. They are not driven or hurried. They live with a sense that there is adequate time to do what needs to be done each day."[8] While the poor may lack many of the conveniences and resources to which I have easy access, they are rich in unhurried time. Perhaps we first-world folks don't realize the true cost of our hurried way.

UNHOLY HURRY IN THE CHURCH?

Even when it comes to the work of ministry, it sometimes appears that the goal is to keep people busy with ministry jobs. In *The Way of the Heart*, Henri Nouwen suggests a different aim: "Our task is to help people concentrate on the real but often hidden event of God's active presence in their lives. Hence, the question that must guide all organizing activity in a parish is not how to keep people busy, but how to keep them from being so busy that they can no longer hear the voice of God who speaks in silence."[9] And it is hearing the voice of God in the quiet that enables us to live and work well. Instead of being a guarantee of fruitfulness, overwork can become a guarantee against it.

Yet Nouwen's words can sound like the antithesis of many of our church and ministry experiences. Whenever we can, we should seek to develop a Christian culture that provides us with enough unhurried time that we can be attentive to the voice of God. Unhurry enables us to notice God's very real but often hidden activity around us, among us and in us. Extended times to be alone and quiet with God tune me back in to reality. I keep thinking that "real" life is all the tasks and emails and bills and projects and other things that fill my schedule. But Jesus himself is real life. And real life in Jesus is eternal and spacious, not condensed, compressed, compacted. Real life is huge and unhurried. Hurry constricts my world, making it much narrower and smaller. And as hurry narrows my vision, I lose perspective on what matters most.

As I think along these lines, I wonder about those people who have expressed disappointment in their years of busyness—their years of faithfully laboring at what they were told would result in their maturity and spiritual growth, only to find that they were more busy than they were rooted in Christ and growing in him. Such dissatisfaction is evidence that there wasn't much spiritual life in their efforts. One pastor admits, "Seeing crowds of people coming together to seek Jesus gives me great joy. . . . But does this business, this busyness, mean I'm a successful pastor? Maybe it does, but maybe it doesn't. It may indicate that I have a problem."[10]

Sometimes the problem at the root of our overwork is the fact that many of us only feel comfortable when we are *doing* something. But *doing* and *fruitfulness* are not necessarily synonyms. Gerald May shares this observation:

> Today many of us have been [so] conditioned by efficiency that times [of sitting on the porch] feel unproductive, irresponsible, lazy, even selfish. We know we need rest, but we can no longer see the value of rest as an end in itself; it is only worthwhile if it helps us recharge our batteries so we can be even more efficient in the next period of productivity.[11]

Many of us only feel valuable when we are checking something off our to-do list. We therefore struggle to enter into the gift of rest as a good in itself.

As I suggest in chapter seven, good work grows best in the soil of good rest. This seems to me the best sequence. My own overwork has a hollow, unrooted quality about it. I think I'm getting a lot done, but my progress is more like running in circles than making a graceful journey of significance.

Thomas Merton, the Trappist prophet of the last century, made this important contribution to a discussion of work:

The fact that our works are done in the service of God is not enough, by itself, to prevent us from losing our interior life if we let them devour all our time and all our strength. Work is good and necessary, but too much of it renders the soul insensitive to spiritual values, hardens the heart against prayer and divine things. It requires serious effort and courageous sacrifice to resist this hardening of heart.[12]

Overwork is heart-hardening. People who are driven, who tend to be workaholics, are more prone to developing atherosclerosis (hardening of the arteries). Such hardening happens to our spiritual hearts as well when we are too busy. But what if we think our work is God's work? What if we find ourselves in the strange neighborhood of "overworking for God"? Why do we do this?

Sometimes we get snared by the belief that we are what we do. What we do is an expression of who we are; what we do does not establish who we are. This reversal of primary identity and secondary identity can energize unhealthy drivenness and be deadly to our soul. Such hyperactivity may produce impressive quantitative results, but the consequent heart-hardening hinders the degree to which the Spirit might energize these efforts. As evidence, consider the common lack of the Spirit's most basic fruit—patience, kindness, peace or gentleness, to name a few—in such leaders' lives.

Do we believe that numeric success is reason enough to disregard the lack of deep spiritual fruit in our lives? Are we willing to settle for obvious, outward success when the chances are slim that God's Spirit is the source of such work and thereby ensuring its lasting fruitfulness?

Thomas Merton talked about those people who never enter into the gift of the more contemplative life that God has for each of us. He explained why that happens:

[These people] are attached to activities and enterprises that seem to be important. Blinded by their desire for ceaseless motion, for a constant sense of achievement, famished with a crude hunger for results, for visible and tangible success, they work themselves into a state in which they cannot believe that they are pleasing God unless they are busy with a dozen jobs at the same time. Sometimes they fill the air with lamentations and complain that they no longer have any time for prayer, but they have become such experts in deceiving themselves that they do not realize how insincere their lamentations are. They not only allow themselves to be involved in more and more work, they actually go looking for new jobs.[13]

I can find myself seeking first work for God rather than God's own kingdom work and righteousness. Instead of the prayer of my heart echoing Jesus' own prayer—"your kingdom come, your will be done"—my prayer sounds more like "Bless where I'm trying to reign and bless what I'm trying to do."

This isn't a new problem, unique to believers in the past couple of centuries. It is said that fourteenth-century philosopher and theologian Catherine of Siena once asked the Lord why he seemed so present to his people in the time of the Scriptures but seemed so absent in her own time. God's answer is as true today as it was then:

[God seemed so present to people in biblical times] because they came to Him as faithful disciples to await His inspiration, allowing themselves to be fashioned like gold in the crucible or painted on by His hands like an artist's canvas, and letting Him write the law of love in their hearts. Christians of [Catherine's] time acted as if He could not see or hear them, and wanted to do and say everything by themselves, keeping themselves so busy and restless that they would not allow Him to work in them.[14]

In the fourteenth century, as in ours, hurry was at least part of the reason why people didn't experience the presence of God.

What about our experience of church today? There seems to be a common assumption that being a more committed Christian will involve an increasing level of programmatic involvement at church (or at least in church programming): weekly worship services, youth or children's ministries, a men's or women's study, a regular small group, service projects and so on. Is it possible that all of this "doing" might need to be undone at some point so that we can make enough open space and unhurried time to enjoy the God we follow, and to hear his invitation to follow him and serve his particular purposes in our lives?

In my work on this "unhurried time" writing project, I continue to see evidence that our hurry, rather than getting *more* done, often gets the wrong thing done—and a lot of it! Christ-followers need to slow down enough to listen to the Master for specifics about what it is that he actually wants.

So how might we envision a life of rich fruitfulness, of true productivity?

GRACED FRUITFULNESS

What does the genuine productivity of holy unhurry look like? I think of Paul's description of his own grace-empowered hard work: "By the grace of God I am what I am, and his grace to me was not without effect. No, I worked harder than all of them—yet not I, but the grace of God that was with me" (1 Cor 15:10). Grace enables quality, hard work. Grace does not inspire fruitless overwork.

Consider this parable. There was once a king who had two servants. One of the servants, for fear of not pleasing his master, rose early each day to hurry along to do all the things that he believed the king wanted done. He didn't want to bother the king with questions about what that work was. Instead, he hurried from project to project from early morning until late at night. The other servant, also eager to please his master, would rise early as well, but he took a few moments to go to the king, ask him about his wishes for the day and find out just what it was he desired to be done. Only after such a consultation did this servant step into the work of his day, work comprised of tasks and projects the king himself had expressed an interest in and a desire for. The busy servant may have gotten a lot done by the time the inquiring servant even started his work, but which of them was doing the will of the master and pleasing him? Genuine productivity is not about getting as much done for God as we can manage. It is doing the good work God actually has for us in a given day. Genuine productivity is learning that we are more than servants, that we are beloved sons and daughters invited into the good kingdom work of our heavenly Father. That being the case, how might God be inviting you to wait for his specific direction? Or is God inviting you to take a specific step now?

I think of a story that one of our Journey alumni shared with me when she was going through our training. The Journey is a process I lead with a team of colleagues for The Leadership Institute. It is a two-year, six-retreat training course that integrates spiritual formation and leadership development for groups of twenty to twenty-five Christian leaders who go through it together. She often found herself leading worship in gatherings of her organization's leaders. In one session, she included two minutes of silence for these national directors of this international ministry to listen for God and reflect on his voice. Not a common practice in these meetings, this silence might have been dismissed by some as a waste of time. But God spoke into the silence.

One of the leaders present, who was responsible for a large ministry in a closed-access nation, had shared how painful and challenging the ministry had been since a severe government crackdown on all Christian ministries. During those two minutes of corporate silence, God gave this leader a strategy for how to move forward in light of those very real challenges. The plan had the aroma of God's grace, was imbued with a sense of his initiative and invitation, and tasted of life and encouragement. Those two minutes of silence— what may well have felt quite counterintuitive for some of the leaders in that gathering—bore the fruit of profound wisdom and divine direction for this leader. Genuine productivity is indeed the fruit of active abiding in Christ.

Do the works of my life demonstrate God's favor toward me and his gracious work in me? Is the pace of my life Christlike? What about my life, if anything, would press another to admit, "What you are doing could only exist if God's favor were with you"? Or is the fruit of my life the result of my busyness and nonstop activity? From which source comes the more lasting fruit? What if I learned to work from a place of unhurried *abiding*? Isn't that what Jesus did? We find no evidence that Jesus was ever in a rush. In fact, there is *more* evidence that at times Jesus frustrated his followers because of his lack of hurry. Jesus lived an unhurried *and* fruitful life. This fact can sound like an oxymoron to us.

UNHURRIED TIME

1. When have you most recently needed to respond without delay to a truly urgent need? Put differently, when has the Spirit most recently invited you into a moment of holy hurry?

2. When has procrastination snuck up on you and tempted you to unholy unhurry? In the moment, what good work—that you realize now was a holy invitation—did you put off?

3. Explain how this book's message about unhurriedness could tempt you to justify places of laziness in your thinking, your intentions, or your way of life and work.

4. In what aspects of your life is acedia a struggle or temptation?

5. In what ways has the temptation to overwork as a means of trying to establish a confident sense of identity become a place of disconnection from fruitful communion with the God of that very work?

4

TEMPTATION

Unhurried Enough to Resist

Mark is the CEO of a large, nationwide company. He is an impressive individual who turns heads when he walks into the room and holds people's attention with his commanding presence. Everybody looks up to him due to his six-foot-plus stature and his influential position. Having risen from humble beginnings, Mark has a real rags-to-riches story. He seems to succeed at everything he tries.

Bob is Mark's wisest and most trusted adviser: he always has the right answer for any situation. Bob is a longtime mentor and a board member of the company Mark leads. Mark doesn't remember ever getting bad advice from him. Many leaders consider him a real business guru, and Mark is very glad Bob is in his corner. Mark met Bob when he was just out of college and trusts him without question. Theirs is a sort of father-son relationship, but that relationship is currently being tested.

Mark's company is in the process of completing what could be the biggest deal in its history, but they are up against a much larger, multinational company. Getting the details right is critical. A wrong move would be fatal. There is no room for missteps.

Very aware of that fact, Bob tells Mark that he needs to do some more research on the deal. He has some misgivings about certain

details and urges Mark to hold off doing *anything* for a week until
he's back in touch. Mark is to take no action and sign no papers
until Bob does his due diligence. "Trust me," Bob urges, and Mark
agrees reluctantly. After all, he's the CEO, the decision maker, and
he feels a little hamstrung by Bob's counsel.

As the week wears on, Mark's stress level rises. The larger company's presence is menacing and worrisome; the potential deal may
be unraveling. Mark tries to reach Bob, but he doesn't answer his
cell phone. Nor does he respond to texts, voicemails, emails—
nothing! Mark becomes more and more agitated, and everyone in
the office is walking on eggshells. A week later, to the day, Mark
still hasn't heard a thing from Bob. He's frustrated and indignant.
From his perspective, the deal is in jeopardy. Something must
be done. Action needs to be taken. Bob has delayed too long. No
matter what he's discovered while working on the deal this past
week, that information won't matter at all if the other company is
as close to signing a contract as they seem to be.

So Mark makes a couple of calls, pulls the trigger and makes
the deal. He feels relieved and triumphant—and furious that Bob
failed to get back to him. He can't wait to fill Bob in on the amazing
deal when he finally decides to show up. Suddenly—and within
moments of the phone call that closed the deal—Bob walks into
Mark's office. "Friend, be glad I took the time I did to take a closer
look into this opportunity. Everything wasn't what it appeared. On
closer investigation, the details didn't add up. The proposed deal
is a disaster waiting to happen, and whoever gets stuck with it is
going to wish they hadn't. There's no way we want any part of this
thing. We need to drop it—and drop it now!"

When Mark's jaw drops, Bob wonders what's going on. "I already
made the call. The deal was slipping away. The other company was
sweetening its offer, threatening to win the contract, so I made the
call and did the deal."

Bob explodes: "What were you thinking? *Were* you thinking? You've jeopardized the entire company! When news gets out of just how bad this deal really is, our stock price is going to drop right through the floor. The board is going to have your head, Mark. Your days are definitely numbered."

SAUL AND SAMUEL

Maybe that situation reminds you of the Old Testament account of King Saul and his adviser, Samuel. Saul's business is serving the nation of Israel as king, and Samuel is a prophet of the Lord, a wise and trusted consultant for the king. Samuel tells Saul to wait, promising to come and make an offering to the Lord on Israel's behalf (1 Sam 13:8). Saul does wait the seven days but, in the face of imminent danger and plummeting troop morale, gives in to temptation and makes the offering himself. Only moments later Samuel arrives, one week later, just like he promised. Instead of trusting that God's prophet would keep his word and walking the path God had for him, Saul took action. His decision to offer the sacrifice himself cost him his leadership of the nation of Israel—quite a price for hurry. Scripture contains many other tragic stories about people who succumbed to the temptation to hurry ahead of God's plan or in a different direction in hopes of reaching the same destination sooner.

Hurrying to act can come with a cost—often a high cost, as it did for Saul. Yet slowing down isn't easy. Our culture values quick decision making in leaders. To-do lists are long, even never-ending, and busyness can be a status symbol of sorts. Yet none of these values reflects our Lord's way of life when he walked this planet.

Consider, for instance, what Jesus did when he learned about Lazarus's serious illness. Was the Jesus who heard about his close friend and waited two days before going to him hurried or unhurried? Was the Jesus who responded to the bleeding woman's needs when Jairus's daughter was near death hurried or unhurried?

Jesus was engaged and active, but unanxious and unhurried.

Is the God who waited twenty-five years to fulfill his promise and give Abraham a son hurried or not? Impatient hurry is what drove Abraham and Sarah to attempt to help God keep his promise by orchestrating—as those in their culture often did—the birth of Ishmael through Hagar. A God for whom a day is as a thousand years is *not* in a hurry (2 Pet 3:8).

Hurry is a great temptation. Hurry looks like impulsive, knee-jerk reactions: "I'll act now because I may never have another chance!" The temptation to hurry is fueled by the lie that the only good to be had must be grabbed now or never. Jesus' encounter with the devil in the wilderness right after his baptism at the Jordan illustrates the hurried nature of temptation and a holy response to it. Jesus is a master of the unhurried response to tempting suggestions.

LED IN THE FULLNESS OF THE SPIRIT

Jesus has just heard his Father's affirming words at his baptism: "You are my Son, whom I love; with you I am well pleased" (Lk 3:22). Then we are told that he is "led by the Spirit into the wilderness" (Lk 4:1). Now, here in the desert, the tempter seeks to turn God's statement into a question. Where God puts a period (or even an exclamation mark), the tempter puts a question mark. He adds an *if* to God's faithful promises. He wants to turn God's gifts into something we deserve, we need to earn, or we must trick God into giving us. Can you imagine gifts under the Christmas tree with price tags like that on them?

The Spirit leads Jesus on a forty-day sojourn in the desert where he is tempted by the devil. If you, like Jesus, had waited until you were thirty to begin your ministry, wouldn't you have expected to start with different steps? Again we see that God's ways are not our ways. We must learn to follow Jesus' way rather than our own. And, yes, Jesus enters into forty days of disengagement despite waiting until he was thirty years old to start ministering. He was unhurried.

When we think about being led by God's Spirit, do we expect that path to take us into the wilderness? I don't think so. More often we expect the exact opposite: to be taken to an oasis of blessing, comfort and ease. Yet the Spirit leads Jesus into trial, discomfort and difficulty. Forty days like that do not pass quickly. Those days are unhurried—and unhurried isn't necessarily a relaxed paradise.

As we know, during those forty days of fasting in the wilderness, Jesus is tempted by the devil, and I believe we can read those temptations as the devil's attempt to hurry Jesus along. The tempter wants Jesus to consider getting what he needs and doing what he is called to do in his own timing: "Get at it! Get what you need! Do what God told you to do! Make it happen! What are you waiting for?" But Jesus *resists* the temptation to hurry. Amazing—and an amazing example for us!

Jesus' fasting amplifies the unhurried nature of that wilderness journey. Whenever I've fasted for a more extended time (never for forty days, though), I have moved slower by necessity: my bodily systems have slowed due to lack of food. That slowing has helped me pay better attention to spiritual realities than when my body is swimming (drowning?) in calories.

It's no surprise, then, that we often fight our greatest battles with temptation when we are lonely and isolated or feeling needy—and being hungry qualifies! We see from Jesus' wilderness experience that he knows how to resist temptation, even when he is at his weakest. We also see that Jesus knows who to worship and obey, as well as what to invest his life in and what to avoid. Yet making those right choices is often difficult. No wonder we're tempted to see God's leading of us into the wilderness as evidence of his diminished care, but at those times we can know profound fellowship with him, heightened sensitivity to his voice and deeper reliance on his strength.

Someone has contrasted the temptation of Adam and the temptation of Jesus: Adam gave in to temptation even though he had not fasted forty days, but Jesus, who had fasted, stood strong against the tempter. Adam was in a garden, but Jesus was in a wilderness. Adam had access to the fruit of any tree in the garden except one, but Jesus had no food. Jesus was tested when he was at a point of extreme physical weakness, but despite this disadvantage, he resisted.

The tempter uses three specific schemes to call the Father's care into question and to provoke a rash reaction from Jesus. In his response Jesus can teach us how to resist our enemy's false promises and cling to the truth of his way.

TEMPTATION #1: GRAB WHAT YOU NEED

> The devil said to him, "If you are the Son of God, tell this stone to become bread." Jesus answered, "It is written: 'Man shall not live on bread alone.'" (Lk 4:3-4)

With each of the temptations, the devil seeks to plant uncertainty in Jesus' heart about his calling and his identity. The devil likes to say "if" where God makes solid promises. The evil one seeks to plant doubt and uncertainty when God would have us know peaceful, confident unhurry. The enemy tempts us to run when we should be waiting.

> Devil: "You're hungry, Jesus. Act *now* and make yourself a meal from these stones!"
>
> Jesus: "Bread isn't everything, and it isn't what I need most. I'll trust my Father to provide what I need most when he is ready to provide it."

The devil tempts Jesus to make provision for himself here and now.

Likewise, our enemy tempts us to hurry ahead of God's provision.

In his book *Three Mile an Hour God*, theologian Kosuke Koyama suggests why this "man does not live by bread alone" lesson was significant to the children of Abraham as they were in a wilderness hundreds of years before Jesus was in one: "Before they went into the land of Canaan, God decided to spend forty years to teach this one lesson. Mind you, forty years for one lesson! How slow and how patient."[1] Temptation leads us to be in too big a hurry to learn the lessons in patience and trust that God wants his children to master. After all, God himself isn't in a hurry because he's seeking to do quality work.

Yet in the garden, the devil insinuated that God was taking his sweet time to fulfill the deep needs of Adam and Eve's souls, that God was holding out on them and they needed to grab for the gusto. Such grabbing is not a holy choice. It is a fall into temptation and a step away from communion with God. Adam and Eve grabbed for an opportunity to be like God—and they lost the gift of an open, intimate relationship with God. They were tempted to act apart from the Father to get what they believed they needed now. Yielding to that temptation revealed their doubt that God would keep his promise and provide what they needed. Not showing much creativity, the tempter revisits this theme with Jesus. His unchanging methods have been very effective for a long time.

Again, hurry is impulsive, a knee-jerk reaction revealing an "I'm gonna act now because I may never have another chance" mindset. Temptation seeks to shrink the time between impulse and action. (Compulsive and addictive living allows no time between impulse and action.) In contrast, wisdom calls us to be discerning about our impulses and inclinations. Are they prompted by God's Spirit? Are they the Spirit's leading? Or do they have another source?

Another way to think about this "bread alone" insight is that we're in such a hurry because we tend to define ourselves by what we have—and the more we have, the more valuable we are. "British preacher Campbell Morgan once said that persecution was the devil's second-best tactic. His best tactic is materialism, and we in the West have been sleepwalkers in our faith for too long, forgetting in the midst of a life of material ease and manic busyness that we are even in a spiritual battle."[2] We find ourselves working harder to earn more money to buy more and more things that we don't really need. This cycle accelerates our lives. Put differently, temptation encourages us to buy into this false equation: "Possessing more + consuming more = living more." Succumbing to this temptation traps us in busyness, and we have walked into that trap without even recognizing it. Maybe the following analogy will help us look more discerningly at our lives.

Imagine a Christmas scene where the kids come into the living room and begin frantically grabbing their gifts, tearing them open ungratefully. They miss the joy of gratitude. They lose the pleasure of giving and receiving. Gratitude is one gift that gets squeezed out when we let materialism speed up our lives. Materialism sees gratitude as inefficient, diminishing our opportunity to take credit for achievements and accomplishments that God has enabled.

We are to resist this temptation by doing what Jesus did. We choose to remember that life is about much more than food (or shelter, clothes or other possessions). Life is learning to abide in an eternal reality. We human beings are truly alive when we let ourselves be nourished by God, satisfied by God and sustained by God. Temptation would claim that waiting for these is a waste of time.

Shirley Carter Hughson, an Anglican Benedictine abbot from the last century, suggested that "in trying to dedicate every moment to God, just remember that the time of waiting, doing nothing as the world would say, is just as much an offering to God as hours of prayer or work. Even puritanic Milton realized that 'they also serve who only stand and wait.' Do not let Satan tempt you to be in a hurry about anything."[3]

TEMPTATION #2: TAKE CHARGE!

The devil led him up to a high place and showed him in an instant all the kingdoms of the world. And he said to him, "I will give you all their authority and splendor; it has been given to me, and I can give it to anyone I want to. If you worship me, it will all be yours." Jesus answered, "It is written, 'Worship the Lord your God and serve him only.'" (Lk 4:5-8)

Devil: "You've been announcing the kingdom is *near*. Well, I can make all these kingdoms of the world yours *right now* if you just worship me!"

Jesus: "Not a chance, Satan. I worship and serve God alone. He will reveal his kingdom and give me authority in his good timing."

The devil is saying that Jesus can get authority *now*. No need to wait. No need to suffer. No need for the cross. We can do this *now!* The strategy is simple. The evil one tempts us to hurry ahead of God and his timetable for giving authority and bestowing honor. We want power and influence. We want to shine. We want to be lifted up in the eyes of others. We want to be noticed. All of these come as grace-gifts from the Father, not as prizes to be earned. Legitimate authority and genuine honor are *always* given. So the temptation is to seize power rather than waiting to receive it from God's hand in God's time and in God's way. Temptation says, "Everything is out there for the taking." God, in his grace, says that everything is there to be received and shared.

The devil tempts Jesus to do what the Father was calling him to do—to rule over the kingdoms of the world—but to do it in his own timing and his own way, rather than trusting God to guide him in his perfect timing and his perfect way.

What bait did the devil put on his hook? He told Jesus, "You can rule over all kingdoms now"—and the kingdoms of this world are indeed subject to the tempter's influence. What was the hook? "Worship me to gain authority over those kingdoms." Like every temptation the liar presents, this offer has elements of both truth and falsehood. The tempter could claim to have a great deal of power and authority in the world, but he could not claim to be sovereign over all the world. His offer is oversell, if not an outright lie.

So what is the bait that the devil uses to tempt us? "You can make a difference and have an impact right now and on your own." The hook? "Just do things *for* God. Don't wait or worry about doing them *with* God."

What was the Father's way to give the Son all authority in heaven and on earth? It was the way of suffering (Phil 2:5-11). Can we, his followers, expect our path to be any different?

How do we resist the temptation to grab glory for ourselves? We keep our focus on God. We honor him. We humble ourselves, trusting that, when he's ready, God will lift us up. Lifting *ourselves* up is physically impossible and spiritually unwise. True influence is always given to us by God; it is not something we take for ourselves.

TEMPTATION #3: PROVE THAT GOD CARES!

The devil led him to Jerusalem and had him stand on the highest point of the temple. "If you are the Son of God," he said, "throw yourself down from here. For it is written: 'He will command his angels concerning you to guard you carefully; they will lift you up in their hands, so that you will not strike your foot against a stone.'" Jesus answered, "It is said, 'Do not put the Lord your God to the test.'" (Lk 4:9-12)

Devil: "Why wait to prove that you are the Son of God? A miraculous jump from this temple peak with a flashy rescue from God's angels would prove your identity in a moment."
   Jesus: "Why would I test the Father's timing or provision?"

The evil one tempts us to rush to make a name for ourselves rather than wait to receive the name he has for us. In this third temptation, the evil one questions Jesus' identity—"Does God really care about you?"—and tempts him to prove God's care in a way that everyone will recognize.

The temple, where this temptation occurs, was God's dwelling place. It was a physical representation of the Emmanuel, "God with Us," truth that we celebrate each Christmas. The devil tempts Jesus to leap from the place of God's presence to demonstrate that God's caring presence really is with him. But, in the words of theologian Henri Nouwen, Jesus was unwilling to be a stuntman.[4]

Do you and I sometimes try to do God's *will* but not in God's *way*? The tempter leads us to do this by quoting the Scriptures for his own distorted purposes. There is no magic in claiming Scripture as an authority for our actions. We must be living in submission to the way of Christ if we want to stand strong against the enemy's temptations and live in the life of Christ.

Satan tempts Jesus to test God's protection of him and tries to force him to act. "Make him do what he has promised," the evil one challenges. Satan wants us to treat God's promises as if they are a legal contract rather than as a covenant that seals a loving relationship. I was watching a television minister talk about biblical promises God makes to heal. He said, "I decided that, whether God liked it or not, I was going to make him keep his promise to heal."

What perception of God does that statement suggest?

How do we resist the temptation to test God's care for us or to find our primary identity somewhere other than in him? We choose to *trust* in his care, and as he provides, we come to trust him with more and more of our hearts. You and I benefit when we choose to recall past expressions of God's care when we are struggling in order to see such expressions in the present. May we also choose to let God be the One who declares our worth.

Wait a Minute!

We all sometimes feel that God has delayed the fulfillment of some promise or the answer to our prayer for guidance. Certain events aren't happening for us as soon as we expected or wanted. Maybe we can do something to help God along, we wonder. I remember a season when my wife and I had many leaders encouraging us and affirming that God had plans to expand our ministry. We were serving in a smaller church as ministers to young adults at the time. It was pretty heady stuff. We had people we didn't know and who didn't know each other say the same things about us. We felt a strong and clear sense of confirmation. But months went by and then years. A decade later, any objective bystander would have said that our outward influence had, if anything, decreased. Did we hear wrong? Were all those people mistaken? I've come to believe that we were expecting a skyscraper to be built on the fast track. And in ways disconnected from much intentional effort on my part, new doors for influence have begun to open—nearly twenty years later. I don't think anyone would use the metaphor of a skyscraper to describe our influence yet, but they might say it's increasing.

I find it hard to trust when I have to wait so long for a promise to begin to become a reality. Like Jesus in the desert, I need to learn to abide in a certain word from Scripture that stands as a holy invitation to us when we face temptation: *wait.*

In the decades before his ministry begins and in the forty wilderness days, Jesus is willing to wait, and his example calls us to cultivate that same posture before the Father. Jesus teaches us that there are times when the right response to our circumstances is to wait. The Spirit will lead us to places where we live out our trust in God by waiting, not acting. After all, there are things that God and only God can do in us, for us, through us. And God is the Lord of timing, and his timing is quite good—as in perfect! You and I do not have the expansive perspective that the Father does. We live with a very limited perspective but with a keen awareness of what is squeezing us and tempting us to hurry rather than wait. And hurry has a way of narrowing our perspective even further, giving us a sort of spiritual tunnel vision.

Temptation is unhealthy hurry. Key to this insight is the verb *wait*, a word used often in Scripture to describe an aspect of our relating to God and one that we Americans don't like at all. Hear what God and his people say in Scripture:

> We wait in hope for the LORD;
>> he is our help and our shield.
> In him our hearts rejoice,
>> for we trust in his holy name.
> May your unfailing love be with us, LORD,
>> even as we put our hope in you. (Ps 33:20-22)

Holy unhurry flourishes in a heart full of hope. Its opposite—hopelessness—can cause us to be driven, anxious and frantic. When we wait on God, our vision of his reliability and immense care for us is sharpened. Hurry blurs our vision. When I drive through a beautiful part of the country at freeway speed, I can't make out many details. The same is true if I am zipping through life. A few summers ago, my brother, my dad and I rode our bikes down the Oregon coast, covering about four hundred miles over five days. I saw the landscape at cycle speed rather than rushing past it at freeway speed. The experience was rich and wonderful. A more unhurried pace in life yields many rewards.

> Be still before the LORD
>   and wait patiently for him;
> do not fret when people succeed in their ways,
>   when they carry out their wicked schemes.
> Refrain from anger and turn from wrath;
>   do not fret—it leads only to evil. (Ps 37:7-8)

One temptation to unholy hurry comes when we see others appearing to succeed in their willful, destructive plans. Anger rushes us to judgment and perhaps even to vengeance. Anger is soul hurry. Patience is soul unhurry. Fretting is soul hurry. Peace is a soul unhurried and at rest. I hurry when I believe deep down that God is not watching over and caring for me. I rush to do for myself what I somewhere, deep down, believe God is failing to do for me.

> Yet the LORD longs to be gracious to you;
>   therefore he will rise up to show you compassion.
> For the LORD is a God of justice.
>   Blessed are all who wait for him! (Is 30:18)

The God for whom I wait does not ration out his generosity. He *longs* to be gracious to us. What might it do to the pace of my heart if I were more confident of God's genuine desire to bless me? Would I rush around trying to achieve and grab if I let myself believe that God longs to give me more than I can clutch in my white-knuckled fists?

> I say to myself, "The LORD is my portion;
>   therefore I will wait for him."
> The LORD is good to those whose hope is in him,
>   to the one who seeks him;
> it is good to wait quietly
>   for the salvation of the LORD." (Lam 3:24-26)

Jeremiah speaks to himself, and I've found that this kind of holy talking to myself helps me too. I can remind myself that God is my portion and the One who fills my plate. I can speak to my soul when it behaves like a frantic kid or a hurried adolescent within me. I can remind my soul that God will indeed fill my plate and that he will give me everything I need to really live. Why do I rush through this world as though it were an all-you-can-eat buffet right before the restaurant closes and the serving trays are almost empty? What if I can learn to unhurriedly trust that God himself will fill my plate with all that I need?

One practical form this talking to myself takes is learning to pay attention to my thoughts. This practice has deep roots in the tradition of the desert fathers with their focus on seven (or eight) deadly thoughts. Their focus was more on the thoughts that lead us to sin rather than on the sins themselves. Scripture invites me to "take captive every thought to make it obedient to Christ" (2 Cor 10:5), but that's hard to do if I'm not even noticing my thoughts. When my thoughts are on autopilot rather than manual control, I find myself in places I really didn't want to revisit. Some of my thoughts are my own. Some may be given me by the Spirit. Some may come from my enemy. When I notice my thoughts, paying attention to what I'm actually thinking, I can discern the likely source of these thoughts and decide whether I choose to act on them or resist them.

Recently, as I was preparing to share an early version of one of these chapters with some friends in another country, I was feeling anxious and lacking confidence. I noticed a few thoughts connected with these feelings. *This chapter isn't good enough to read aloud,* and *Reading a book aloud at a conference is a waste of their time,* and *Reading this chapter with translation will be slow and just won't work.* As I noticed these thoughts, it didn't take me long to see in them a discouraging tone that does not come from the Spirit of Jesus. I decided to resist them and move forward with my original plan.

When I went ahead and shared that chapter portion, the outcome was completely different from what those thoughts were predicting. This was further confirmation that I had been guided well by the Spirit to resist them. What thoughts are going through your mind even now? Can you notice them so that you might decide how to sort them out?

Consider one more passage that helps us learn the fruitfulness of waiting on God's presence and timing:

> Be patient, then, brothers and sisters, until the Lord's coming.
> See how the farmer waits for the land to yield its valuable crop,
> patiently waiting for the autumn and spring rains. You too, be
> patient and stand firm, because the Lord's coming is near. Don't
> grumble against one another, brothers and sisters, or you will
> be judged. The Judge is standing at the door! (Jas 5:7-9)

A valuable crop doesn't grow overnight. And we don't always experience the fruit of God's promises as soon as we might prefer. Yes, life is more like farming than a factory production line. In life, we wait because we don't have control of so many of the processes that bring or hinder life—metaphorically speaking, the processes of rain, sun, frost, disease, pests and so on. The land *yields* its crop. Instead of waiting for the fruit to grow, we try to grab the crop from the land.

Consider the story of God's promise to Abraham that he and Sarah would have their own son, one born from their union. He and Sarah are both way too old for this to happen. They see the fulfillment of this promise as impossible. After waiting ten years, Sarah figures that God needs some help keeping his promise, so she suggests Abraham sleep with her maidservant, Hagar, so they can produce the promised child (Gen 16). But that child—named Ishmael and produced by that act of rushing God's timing—becomes the head of a race of people who have been in continual conflict with the people of Israel for countless generations. Abraham's choice to act apart from God instead of waiting on his ways and his timing continues to haunt the people of God and, in fact, the world at large. The price of Abraham's rushed action is difficult to measure. He is a good and tragic example of the truth that "[the one] who is in a hurry delays the things of God."

At this point of your journey, what are the toughest temptations you face? Do you struggle to stand strong against anger? lust? pride? envy? Why might slowing down enable you to recognize the emptiness of these unholy suggestions? And what might you do to see and trust more that God really *does* want to provide for you, even if you feel you've been walking in a barren wilderness for a while now? What might you do to grow your trust that God wants to increase the kingdom impact of your life so that it is a light in this world? What could you do even today to practice relying more on God's great care and protection? I pray that, as you slow down inside, your vision will clear, life will be less of a blur, and you will have eyes that see God's great provision, his holy calling and the measureless love of the Father for you.

Unhurried Time

1. When you think of temptation as a rush to grab for ourselves something God wants to give us as a gift, where do you see such hurry in your own life? How do you want to acknowledge this before God, welcoming his mercy and grace to meet you here?

2. Think of some of the waiting places in your life at this stage of your journey. What temptations do these delays raise for you? How might God be inviting you to wait *with him* as you wait *for* what he might do?

3. Which of the three temptations—those related to provision, to authority or honor, or to doubt of God's care—do you find most troublesome at this stage of your journey? How does Jesus' response to that particular temptation help you here?

Unhurried Enough to Care

I'm sitting at a traffic light in my neighborhood, waiting for the red light to turn. I'm trying to be relaxed and unhurried about my life. Before I have a chance to respond to the light that has just turned green, the person behind me is already on his horn. It happens often enough that my wife and I have given this experience a name—*gronk*. It is a contraction of *green* and *honk*, and it represents the nanosecond of time between the fresh green light in front of us and the angry horn blasting behind us. It is an inflammation of impatience. It is an utter lack of simple kindness. It is chronic and epidemic. And, bottom line, it is unloving.

Maybe this sounds to you like whining. I'm tempted to react: "Hey, gronker! What in the world is so important that my slow reaction time is such an offense to you? Do you have an appointment with the president? Are you trying to get your injured child to the hospital?" (I would understand a good solid gronk in this last case.) Probably not. Instead, that gronk is likely just a habit rooted in the belief that time is money and that hurry, therefore, is always profitable. If hurry gets in the way of love, does hurry go or does love go?

LOVE DOESN'T RUSH

In 1 Corinthians 13, when Paul describes the nature of love and loving, the first trait he lists is patience. Patience is an unhurried virtue, and this first descriptor of love highlights the unhurried nature of love. Patience doesn't give up easily. It doesn't lose its temper quickly. It doesn't quit at the first sign of trouble, rush to judgment or run away from an uncomfortable or difficult situation. Neither does love. The older English word for patience is *long-suffering*, a word that communicates patience is willing to bear with hardship awhile. It does so for love and in care for another.

Historian and social philosopher Eugen Rosenstock-Huessy claimed that "the greatest temptation of our time is impatience, in its full original meaning: refusal to wait, undergo, suffer. We seem unwilling to pay the price of living with our fellows in creative and profound relationships."[1] Love doesn't rush past hard places. Love enables us to listen when we are tempted to react. Love moves us to seek understanding when we feel misunderstood. Love is patient.

Consider, for instance, that the God of the Scriptures is in no hurry to become angry with us. But do you truly believe that he is not quick to lose patience with you? When you imagine God having a human face, is he smiling? Or do you picture him as stern or angry? Does he roll his eyes at your frequent falls? Frankly, my gut image of God is often a pretty impatient one. I expect him to have little patience with my slowness to understand him and follow his ways. He seems quick to lose his temper with me. But if, as Paul said in 1 Corinthians 13, love is patient, then God is patient, and he is patient with me.

Kosuke Koyama, a Japanese theologian of the last century, wrote these wise words about God's pace in this world and his reason for that pace:

God walks "slowly" because he is love. If he is not love he

would have gone much faster. Love has its speed. It is an inner speed. It is a spiritual speed. It is a different kind of speed from the technological speed to which we are accustomed. It is "slow" yet it is lord over all other speed since it is the speed of love. It goes on in the depth of our life, whether we notice or not, whether we are currently hit by storm or not, at three miles an hour. It is the speed we walk and therefore it is the speed the love of God walks.[2]

The speed of love is an organic speed, not a mechanical or technological speed. When it comes to machines and technology, faster is always better. When it comes to love, the same is not true. After all, love has a rather constant speed. It is a slow speed, a spiritual speed. "Hurry up and love someone" just doesn't work. Koyama goes on to say, "Jesus is too slow! We want to run before him. . . . The way of Jesus is too slow, inefficient and painful. Jesus' resourcefulness is love. Ours is money."[3] We want Jesus to step it up, to make things happen at our pace, rather than slowing down our pace to match his. Yet his is a pace of caring and concern, not an arbitrary pace of productivity or so-called efficiency.

TAKE TIME TO CARE

Jesus' familiar story of a Samaritan man who cares for the wounded stranger he encounters on his travels models beautifully for us the unhurried nature of those who slow down enough to care for others.

> "A man was going down from Jerusalem to Jericho, when he was attacked by robbers. They stripped him of his clothes, beat him and went away, leaving him half dead. A priest happened to be going down the same road, and when he saw the man, he passed by on the other side. So too, a Levite, when he came to the place and saw him, passed by on the other side. But a Samaritan, as he traveled, came where the man was; and when he

saw him, he took pity on him. He went to him and bandaged his wounds, pouring on oil and wine. Then he put the man on his own donkey, brought him to an inn and took care of him. The next day he took out two denarii and gave them to the innkeeper. 'Look after him,' he said, 'and when I return, I will reimburse you for any extra expense you may have.'

"Which of these three do you think was a neighbor to the man who fell into the hands of robbers?"

The expert in the law replied, "The one who had mercy on him."

Jesus told him, "Go and do likewise." (Lk 10:30-37)

The priest and Levite may well have been returning from temple service and were concerned about becoming ceremonially unclean. They were about to be engaged in doing God's work and were, perhaps, in a hurry to remain faithful to it. They saw the severely wounded man as a distraction from what they were supposed to do for God. Furthermore, their schedules may have been too full to accommodate a wounded person on the way. Maybe they were hurrying along to their next religious duty.

I try to imagine this story set in the present. Maybe a man is driving from Los Angeles to Las Vegas. Who knows why he's going. It's late at night. He gets off the freeway and ends up a little lost on a side road when a group of bikers comes upon him and decides to have some fun at his expense. They drive him off the road, drag him back to the trunk of his car and demand he open it. They beat the life out of the guy while he begs for mercy. They laugh as they rummage through his trunk and his pockets for anything of value. Finally, they leave him—unconscious—lying on the ground between the car and the road.

A few hours later, a church van full of men is driving along that same stretch of road, and they are late for a retreat. They notice the car on the side of the road. The doors and the trunk are open, and the headlights are barely shining. One guy wonders out loud what's going on, another says he thought he saw something on the ground near the car and the driver says, "We're running late. We can't stop."

Soon a van full of Christian college professors comes upon the stranded car. It's gotten dark, and the academics are engrossed in conversation about their book projects and celebrating the beginning of summer with the long days they can spend writing. On their way to Vegas for a convention and glad for a captive audience as they describe their works-in-progress, they are too distracted to notice the half-dead man lying on the road.

Finally, a guy named Larry drives his old rust-box jalopy down that stretch of road. He's on his way to Vegas for a little distraction. Coming upon the stranded car, he wonders what's going on. Having nothing else to do and no real schedule to keep, Larry pulls off the road, and as he does, his headlights fall upon the bleeding man next to the car.

Larry runs over and sees that the man is in bad shape. He returns to his van, grabs an old first-aid kit and does his best to clean up and bandage the worst of the guy's wounds. He uses his own T-shirt as a tourniquet to stop the bleeding. Larry puts the man into the back seat of his jalopy and keeps driving down the road. He doesn't even think about the blood staining the upholstery.

No hospital. No clinic. Nothing. Where can he get help for this guy? Finally, Larry comes upon an old, rundown motel in the middle of nowhere and gets a room. He puts the guy on the only bed and keeps an eye on him. From there, he calls the police, who soon arrive to get his story. The man, coming in and out of consciousness, spends a restless night in that motel bed. Larry sleeps on the floor.

In the morning, Larry goes to the motel clerk and tells him a little of the story. He takes every last bit of cash in his wallet and says, "This is all I have. I know it's not a lot, but the guy I brought here last night is in bad shape, and I'm afraid to move him right now. Would you let him rest here while I go back home to get a few more things and a little more cash? I promise I'll be back to get this guy and pay whatever I'll owe you then." The clerk asks her manager, and he says okay.

Much more is going on in this story Jesus told than people making excuses for not helping someone in obvious need. This parable is a powerful illustration of how hurry keeps us from stopping or even noticing when God puts a bleeding, hurting, lost, desperate, hopeless soul in our path. We are on the road. We have somewhere to go. We have a full schedule. The needy person along the way is an inconvenience, an interruption. I may complain that loving everyone in the world is impossible, but that's not what Jesus commanded. Our Lord and Savior directs us to care for the person who is actually crossing our path. Proximity provides an opportunity to love.

THE UNEXPECTED HERO

Consider now the hero of Jesus' story—the Samaritan who traveled the deserted and notoriously dangerous road from Jerusalem to Jericho, the road nicknamed the Way of Blood. Jews viewed Samaritans as compromisers and half-breeds who had intermarried with the locals and failed in every way to keep the Jewish race pure. Unfaithful. Contaminated. Unclean. Yet we see evidence of unhurried love in this Samaritan's response to the wounded stranger.

The Samaritan saw the wounded man. The priest and Levite noticed the wounded man, but they didn't let themselves truly *see* him. Love looks long enough to be affected by what it sees. Love doesn't look away from what is hard to see.

The Samaritan had pity on the wounded man. The Jewish leaders who walked by didn't let the reality of the wounded man's situation touch their hearts. They were unwilling to be affected by his condition, much less get involved. The Samaritan was different: he was willing to be affected and willing to act.

The Samaritan went to the wounded man. The priest and Levite didn't. Wouldn't it make sense that the Samaritan had plans for his day just as the two Jewish leaders did? But the Samaritan's agenda for the day didn't keep him from responding with unhurried love to the man in need. Love stops when it encounters human need. Love doesn't just walk by. *He went to him* is very different from *he passed by on the other side.* Love makes time to investigate and to serve.

According to Jewish storytelling tradition, the priest should have been the good guy in this story. Instead, he was heartless and perhaps even fearful. He saw the half-dead man with eyes of judgment and/or fear. Perhaps he was also thinking, *The guy is probably a sinner. He had it coming to him. It's not my place to help.* Instead of going near the wounded man, the priest took a wide path around him. That kind of avoidance is a strategy of hurry. It's one thing to notice someone. That can be done in a moment. Hurry glances. Love gazes and often stays and acts. In sharp contrast to the priest, the Samaritan saw—but he saw not with judgment, but with mercy. He let the broken man's desperate plight touch his heart. He didn't harden his heart toward the man.

The Samaritan bandaged the wounds with oil and wine. The Samaritan sought to comfort and care for the wounded man. He offered more than a basic exam and a quick bandage. He offered intensive care. Love is willing to slow down enough to bear the cost of caring.

The Samaritan carried the man to a nearby inn. The Samaritan took the time to travel from this wilderness location to an inn in a nearby town. Who knows how far away it was or how long it took to get the man there. Love doesn't measure care in terms of time.

The Samaritan took the initiative and acted on this wounded man's behalf. He traveled a journey for the wounded man's sake.

The Samaritan stayed overnight with the man. The Samaritan might have been able to entrust the man to someone else, perhaps a first-century professional caregiver. After examining the wounded man, our hero could have had someone else do the rest—but he didn't. The Samaritan was unhurried enough to stay overnight and care for the man. And staying overnight must have affected his plans. Who, for instance, had been expecting him to arrive that evening? What item on the Samaritan's agenda went undone in the name of his love for a stranger?

The Samaritan gave two days' wages so that the wounded man could rest and recover in a more comfortable place. The Samaritan provided for the man the time he needed to recover from his injuries. Too often I want wounded people around me to hurry up and get better because they are inconveniencing me; I want to get on with my life. But what is God's invitation for a given season of my life? Does what I am so hurried to return to really matter? Is it the Lord's priority for me? Or could regaining or retaining a sense of control over my life be more important to me than loving those around me?

One more detail to consider: in the story, the innkeeper seems nothing more than a bit player. But if I were a hotel owner, would I really want a visitor in such bad shape left behind in one of my rooms? The innkeeper—who may well have had little more than mercenary motives—nevertheless did more for the wounded man than the priest or the Levite.

The Samaritan planned a return trip. He intended to check in on this wounded man to see how his recovery was progressing. The Samaritan was also willing to pay any further expenses the man incurred. He cared enough to find out how the man's recovery was going. The Samaritan was unhurried enough to truly care for others.

When Jesus asked the expert in the law, "Which of these was a neighbor to the man?" he hadn't left any doubt as to the right answer. But the legal expert just couldn't bring himself to admit, "The Samaritan." Instead, he simply said, "The one who showed mercy." *Samaritan* is only a category in the law expert's mind, so he isn't about to admit that a Samaritan would be more virtuous than a Jewish leader. In fact, it's also clear that the legal expert who asked Jesus about the meaning of "loving your neighbor" was more interested in justifying himself than in recognizing and caring for his neighbor.

To Follow or Not to Follow?

Do I choose to learn from and follow the good Samaritan's example? Or instead am I sometimes so hurried in my efforts to accomplish everything on my agenda, even on my *God* agenda, that I don't have time to care for someone in obvious need? You and I have perhaps never encountered this exact scene in our everyday travels, but I know I have chosen to walk on the other side of the path and pass by someone with a real need. Perhaps that person was emotionally wounded or spiritually broken. Did I walk by in order to remain faithful to my agenda for the day? And when have I used my sense of God-work and God-calling as an excuse to avoid the God-opportunity to love that is right in front of my face?

Clearly—and this truth is worth repeating—love is unhurried. And since the greatest commandment is to love God and love others, and if genuine love is patient and unhurried, is our hurried life costing us even more than we realize? Does our hurry force us to miss what matters most in life? As I said earlier, Jesus' greatest commandment remains the primary commandment. Nothing preempts it. Nothing supersedes it. God is love. Period. Are we love? Do we love? Love is the bottom line. Love is what matters most. Love is the primary measure God uses to determine what is valuable and what is worthless. Love lasts. And love requires from us a more unhurried approach to life.

I remember a church magazine article that proclaimed the virtues of hurry by using the athletic term *hustle*. But that seems quite at odds with growing in a lifestyle of unhurried love. The greater need we Christ-followers have is to walk at his pace. We want the activity of our lives to bear the holy and rich fruit of communion with Christ. May we avoid the kind of frantic busyness that bears little resemblance to the pace and focus of Jesus' life and ministry.

We don't have to try to figure out how to live at this pace alone. As I think about loving God unhurriedly, John 1:10-11 comes to mind: "He was in the world, and though the world was made through him, the world did not recognize him. He came to that which was his own, but his own did not receive him." Jesus made the world, but the world did not recognize him. Jesus embraced the world, but he was not embraced in return. So am I recognizing Jesus' presence in my daily journey? Am I receiving him as the One who is the way, the truth and the life, or am I so driven by my own agenda that I am running right past his open arms?

When we hear the phrase *receiving Jesus* with our evangelical ears, do we think of an event that occurred at some specific moment in the past? Or do we recognize in that phrase his invitation to an ongoing, unhurried relationship with him? Put differently, do we approach receiving Jesus as a religious transaction or a loving embrace?

I find within myself a deep longing both to enjoy God's embrace and to embrace him in return. I want to slow down enough inside to notice his work and to welcome it. I want to know the vital reality of his presence in my life as I learn to live at the pace of grace. Yet my Christian experience tempts me to think of becoming a Christian as an event in the past rather than a lifelong journey with

God. So I long to sharpen my awareness of him. I need God to heal my dullness, my deafness and my blindness to him.

Near the end of his life, author Henri Nouwen said, "My whole life I have been complaining that my work was constantly interrupted, until I discovered the interruptions were my work."[4] In our hurry, we run right past God-invitations and God-opportunities without even realizing it. We rush to do things for God at such a pace as to miss the appointments his Spirit puts right in front of our noses. I'm guessing that every day we miss opportunities to live a Christlike life, to offer simple expressions of care, affirmation, encouragement and recognition to people who cross our paths. We are moving too fast to stop and act and love.

In fact, I've discovered—and was recently reminded on a trip to another country—that relationships grow best in unhurried time. As I write these paragraphs, I have just finished leading a four-day retreat for Christian leaders in the Dominican Republic. Built into this retreat was a four-hour block of solitude and silence, quite a stretch for this very communal culture. But the unhurried time helps them be more aware that God is with them. I witnessed how this time opened their eyes to one another in love. They became a community without any effort to build community; it was simply the fruit of unhurried communion with God. They didn't seek community first; they sought God, and a richer sense of community resulted, unexpected but very welcome.

Love is patient. Love is slow-paced. Relationships—our relationship with God and our relationships with others—flourish in unhurried time. I've discovered that setting aside some part of one day a month to simply *be* with God enables me to know and rely more on his love for me. This awareness, now deeper in my soul, causes my life to be a cup overflowing, and I'm able to love others from that overflow.

I've also discovered that unhurried time with my wife, Gem,

enriches our care for each other. When all of our interactions are hurried and functional, and only rarely playful or spontaneous, caring seems to fade from them. So we occasionally set aside some part of a day to take a long walk, sit together at the beach, enjoy an unhurried meal or take a leisurely drive. We don't have any critical agenda. We're just together. We talk. We listen. We don't rush things. We're not *making* something happen. We're *receiving* whatever happening God wants to bring our way. We're trying to keep our eyes, our ears, our hearts open to the good things God has been preparing for that moment.

GET OFF THE FREEWAY

I will always remember one particular incident of listening to God and slowing my pace. I was on my way to my office from seminary class. It was a day full of appointments during the season of life when I was trying to be a full-time student and a full-time pastor at the same time. (I still struggle sometimes with the illusion that I can become omnipresent.) With my hour-long drive almost done and my exit only a few miles away, I heard in my heart, "Get off the freeway." *Where did that come from? God, is that you? I have work to do and appointments to keep at the church.* Despite that initial reaction, I responded and took the next off-ramp, a barren and undeveloped exit. My only choice was to turn left at the base of the ramp, where I saw a car with its hood up under the freeway. It was the only vehicle there, but no one could see it. I asked the driver if I could help. He thought perhaps his battery was dead. I had cables in my trunk and was able to get his engine started. Neither of us could have been more grateful for that moment. Unhurry enabled me to care for a neighbor in need. Was anything at the office more important than that?

Though not always that unusual, we are being given opportunities to extend care to another all the time. Perhaps God is inviting *us* to get off the freeway. There are likely good opportunities right under our noses if only we are slow enough to notice them. What we define as interruptions as we hurry along we may come to see as opportunities to love when we go through life at a walking pace. Unhurry helps us loosen our grip on control just enough to start noticing these opportunities. Put differently and more pointedly—and I'm asking myself as well—could we be running past the work God is giving us because we have a hurried, narrow vision of what we're "supposed" to be doing?

THE IDOL OF EFFICIENCY

One of my personal tendencies is to overemphasize efficiency in my approach to living, relating and working. I too often find that my over-the-top focus on efficiency tends to keep me from obeying the great command to love God fully and to love my neighbor freely. I think of the words of Gerald May: "Some people are so caught up in striving for efficiency that love seems like a luxury or even an obstacle to efficient functioning. Taken far enough, this makes for the ominous prospect of people who are very unloving and very efficient at what they do."[5] I surely don't want to be known as unlovingly efficient: "Wow, that guy sure gets things done, even if he doesn't really seem to care about anyone but himself!" Relationships can be messy and not very efficient, but loving relationships are at the heart of the gospel. In the language of efficiency, love is willing to waste time.

For example, I tend to be a very time-conscious person. I prefer to be on time or early for a meeting or appointment. It's a deeply rooted efficiency orientation. My wife is far more relaxed when it comes to these things. Countless times over years of marriage I'll be ready to leave, will know that if we don't leave now we will be late to an event and will begin to think some very unloving thoughts about her. I care more about being faithful to an event's arbitrary

starting time—an event that I am not leading but just attending—
than I care about my partner in life. "My way is virtuous. Her way
isn't." Not very loving, is it? This ticking clock inside of me has a
way of distracting me from a deeper and truer care of people.

Consider the unthinkable triumph of efficiency over love in the
sickening accounts of Nazi middle managers during World War II:
these men took great pride in being able to improve the functioning
of the gas chambers and thus accelerate the extermination rate.
They were somehow able to rationalize in their minds that there
was value in a job "well done," a job they "cared about," even if
that job was killing people. On a much smaller scale, in what way
does our hurry harm others instead of helping them?[6]

I've discovered that when I'm obsessed with efficiency, love feels
like it gets in the way of my reaching that goal. How many of us are
very efficient in managing tasks but very unloving toward the
people whom those tasks involve? If love is patient but my way of
living the Christian life isn't, don't I have a root-level problem here?
How can I live a deeply Christian life without patience or kindness?
Our hearts desperately need to be awakened to the importance of
obeying the Great Commandment, even when obedience seems to
be the most inefficient option. Sometimes ministry positions and
ministry tasks hurry us past ministry opportunities. As I asked
earlier, are we running past and not even seeing the work God is
giving us to do because we have a hurried, narrow vision of what
we imagine is his will for our work?

"As we are increasingly caught by love," May observes, "our usual
standards of efficiency will take a beating. . . . There are points where
I may need to become a little less job-efficient if I want to be more
loving."[7] What if I had to lower my personal standards of productivity in order to be more loving? Would I be willing? If my identity
is based on how well I do or how much I produce, won't that fact
create an immense disincentive to living an unhurried, loving life?

When the kind of hurry we are describing here becomes chronic and obsessive, it may become full-blown hurry sickness. In *Subversive Spirituality*, Paul Jensen mentions three kinds of time pathologies and describes their effects:

- *Time pressure* is the sense that there just isn't enough time for our task or tasks.

- *Time urgency* arises when time pressure becomes a more frequent experience, prompting us to feel the need to hurry or accelerate the rate at which we do things.

- *Hurry sickness* occurs when time urgency has become severe and chronic, changing one's personality and lifestyle.[8]

Jensen points out that these time pathologies have a detrimental effect on relationships in that "it takes time to build and sustain healthy relationships. Time pressures can erode the quality of relationships and create fragmentation and isolation."[9] Hurry creates a false crisis in which I cannot care for the one before me. Instead of being one whose heart is filled by the love of God so that it overflows to others, those other people become a barrier to the ill-defined good I am racing toward. Is my neighbor an obstacle or an opportunity?

If loving my neighbor is an opportunity, then I would benefit from learning the art of lingering. Every couple of weeks, we get together with another couple for unhurried dinner and conversation. It's lingering time. We don't have a minute-by-minute agenda. We aren't trying to complete a Christian checklist. We just enjoy dinner, share our lives, talk about what is helping or hindering us, and linger together in God's presence. We're open to whatever nudges we may sense from God's Spirit. These are good times, even if we don't come away with something we planned for before the dinner began.

As I'm writing this draft in my home office, I look out and see a line of seagulls flying by. They don't seem to be rushing frantically to some next engagement. They dip and glide like they are playing in the breeze. They seem carefree and unhurried. Can I live my life with a little more play and perhaps discover the surprise that I'm also living with a little more love? The pace of my life often feels much less like a playful breeze and much more like a hurricane. Is Jesus inviting me to live that kind of tumultuous life? Does he want my anxiety to rise to such destructive levels? Is my whirlwind of God-activities inspired by God?

Maybe living a little less hurried would enable me each day to notice God-given opportunities to love, opportunities that I am now racing past. Perhaps there are simple moments when I could share a word or gesture of care, but I'm missing them as I focus on getting to the next important item on my full agenda. Love is patient. Am I patient? Love is kind. What about me?

UNHURRIED TIME

1. What is Jesus' answer to the legal expert's question "What must I do to inherit eternal life?" (Lk 10:25-27)? Talk to Jesus about this greatest of commandments. How is he wanting to grow you in enjoying and practicing them?

2. Read Jesus' story of the good Samaritan again (Lk 10:30-37). This time, consider who you most identify with. Jesus? The priest or Levite? The half-dead man? The Samaritan? Imagine the story from that character's perspective. What do you notice from that angle? What impresses you? Where in the story do you think God wants to meet you? Explain.

3. Jesus offers the legal expert a very simple word of counsel: "Go and do likewise" (v. 37). Talk to Jesus about what it would look like for you, in your current circumstances, to go and do the kind of thing the Samaritan did for this broken man. To whom

does Jesus draw your attention? How might he want you to care for that person?

4. The expert in the law asked Jesus to define *neighbor* (v. 29). Perhaps he wanted to argue about it. What is Jesus' answer to his question? What about Jesus' answer impresses you, instructs you and/or helps you?

5. In verse 37, what primary word does the legal expert use to answer Jesus' question about who was the good neighbor? What does this word mean for your life, your relationships and your ministry in this season?

UNHURRIED ENOUGH TO PRAY

It's 4:45 a.m. and my alarm goes off. I'm not usually up at this hour. Sometimes I've risen this early to get in some exercise before a long workday or to avoid Los Angeles traffic if I have a long commute. But today I'm doing an experiment: I'm following Jesus' example. We read in Mark 1:35 that "very early in the morning, while it was still dark, Jesus got up, left the house and went off to a solitary place, where he prayed." I'm awake well before sunrise. Check. I've got a nearby solitary place in mind where I can pray. Check.

I drive to the top of a nearby street and then hike farther to the crest of the hill. I set up my beach chair facing east toward the Santa Ana Mountains, barely outlined against the pretwilight sky. Saddleback Mountain looms before me. The air is cool but not too cold. My light sweatshirt is enough. I hear the chirps of birds and drone of critters in the scrub around me. I hear the occasional call of an owl in a nearby tree. I find myself feeling a little nervous about whether a coyote might come by. And, even at this early hour, I begin to hear many commuters making their way toward the freeway. They're up early for their own reasons.

When I planned this experiment, I wanted to be facing east because I love the sunrise. I won't see it this morning because it's overcast. My iPad lets me access the Bible in the dark as well as journal my thoughts and feelings. (Is this an advantage over Jesus? I doubt it.)

As I read again in Mark 1 about Jesus' rising early to pray, I realize that his day before had been a Sabbath day full of ministry. He had preached in the Capernaum synagogue with authority that surprised the congregation. He had spent the day at Simon and Andrew's home, healed Simon's mother-in-law, and continued healing the sick and delivering the possessed well after sunset. I would have been exhausted. I might very well have slept in the next morning, but Jesus didn't. Communion with his Father mattered so deeply that he rose early enough to have some uninterrupted time to linger with him. It's a good thing Jesus did, because it wasn't long after sunrise that his disciples rushed to bring urgent news that the crowds were looking for him to heal and deliver them and their loved ones. Preaching-healing-delivering became a pattern of Jesus' activity in all the villages of Galilee. It wouldn't surprise me to find that predawn prayer was part of his pattern as well.

All of this makes me want to live the way Jesus lived. But what if following him is about more than just doing the kinds of things he did in ministry—speaking kingdom truth, expressing kingdom love and demonstrating kingdom power? What if following Jesus is also about living life in relationship with the Father just as Jesus himself did? When I think about how Jesus often got away to quiet places to enjoy the presence of his Father, I'm drawn to follow Jesus there too.

What would happen if our following Jesus included his habit of withdrawing often to give the Father his full attention? Would we learn to live Jesus' own unhurried rhythm of life and work? Would we become people who model the life Jesus invites us to know? In Matthew 11:29-30, for instance, he said, "Walk with me and work with me—watch how I do it. Learn the unforced rhythms of grace.

I won't lay anything heavy or ill-fitting on you. Keep company with me and you'll learn to live freely and lightly" (*The Message*). Would we live like that?

Consider this point made by W. F. Adams, C. S. Lewis's spiritual director for a season:

> We can advance along the road to perfection only by walking closely with [Jesus]. And as we watch His way of dealing with the countless problems and troubles that beset His life, we achieve wisdom as to how to meet our own. But to walk with Jesus is to walk with a slow, unhurried pace. Hurry is the death of prayer and only impedes and spoils our work. It never advances it.[1]

In chapter five, we saw that a more unhurried pace of life could help us better love those around us. In this chapter, I want to explore the idea that such unhurry might also help us more fully love the Father through unhurried and conversational prayer.

WHAT GETS JESUS UP IN THE MORNING?

I long to be a person who lives in ever-deepening communion with God. In fact, I believe the desire for that communion is the deepest hunger in every heart, whether acknowledged or not. In Mark 1:35, I see Jesus being very intentional about his relationship with God the Father. But his own followers didn't understand his priorities, and they interrupted him with the urgent demands and expectations of the crowd around them.

Certain things get me up early. Sometimes it's anxiety about a project that is due and not near completion. Sometimes it's an ill-defined drivenness to produce more, possess more, accomplish more, whatever the more may be. I'm the early bird grabbing for the worm before anyone else gets a chance. But Jesus seemed more interested in rising early to focus on the Father and on *his* work. This passion got Jesus up early. The disciples, on the other hand, were more moved by the expectations of the crowd. For them, the crying needs of the crowd seemed to drown out the Father's quiet invitation.

Luke tells us, "At daybreak, Jesus went out to a solitary place" (Lk 4:42). As we've seen, Jesus seemed to have a habit of beginning his day alone with his Father in prayer. I find myself wondering why, having called myself a follower of Jesus for so many years, that habit hasn't been mine as well. I don't say this in guilt or shame, but in sadness and longing. My sense of following Jesus has tended to be more focused on some vague idea of following his moral example or his work of teaching and caring for others. I haven't often thought in practical ways about following his rhythm of life in relation to his Father, the One he taught his first followers to address as *Abba*.

As Luke continues telling Jesus' story, he mentions that he "often withdrew to lonely places and prayed" (Lk 5:16). Despite a life full of ministry responsibilities and opportunities, Jesus practiced a pattern of disengagement in order to be with the Father. Luke uses the word *often*. He didn't say that Jesus chose this early-morning communion with the Father once, or here and there, or on occasion. This consistent prayer time was a regular part of Jesus' daily life when he walked this earth. He practiced this regular rhythm of holy *dis*engagement in the midst of even his busiest seasons of ministry *engagement*. Jesus often withdrew to quiet places where, away from other people, he could give the Father his full and focused attention. Jesus wanted and needed such time with the Father. How life-giving might that same pattern be for us?

If Luke were to describe my pattern of life as he described Jesus', what would that sentence look like? "Alan rarely withdrew to lonely places and prayed" would describe many seasons. What

about you? Would *rarely, occasionally* or *here and there* best describe your pattern? That pattern can change, and this truth may
help motivate you. In these moments of regular retreat in Jesus'
life, he experienced the love of the Father and loved him back.
Alone with *Abba*, Jesus lived in the intimacy that comes with
obeying the great command to love. When I slow down and make
time to be alone with God, I am able to follow Jesus to such places
of communion and fellowship with the Father. May his Spirit em-
power me to slow down enough to wait in God's presence!

Jesus' pattern here is not superhuman. We can actually follow
his example. If we feel we're too busy to follow Jesus in this way,
perhaps we have made ourselves too busy. Jesus came to show us
what a deeply rooted relationship of communion with the Father
could look like, and I believe that the depth of his roots in this vital
and divine relationship is one reason for the broad reach of his influence and for the fruitfulness of his life and ministry.

Consider Henri Nouwen's insight:

> In the midst of a busy schedule of activities—healing suf-
> fering people, casting out devils, responding to impatient dis-
> ciples, traveling from town to town, and preaching from syn-
> agogue to synagogue—we find these quiet words: "*In the
> morning, long before dawn, he got up and left the house, and
> went off to a lonely place and prayed there.*" The more I read
> this nearly silent sentence locked in between the loud words
> of action, the more I have the sense that the secret of Jesus'
> ministry is hidden in that lonely place where he went to pray,
> early in the morning, long before dawn. . . . In the lonely
> place Jesus finds the courage to follow God's will and not his
> own; to speak God's words and not his own; to do God's work
> and not his own. It is in the lonely place, where Jesus enters
> into intimacy with the Father, that his ministry is born.[2]

WHAT KEPT JESUS UP AT NIGHT?

"After leaving them, he went up on a mountainside to pray. Later that night, the boat was in the middle of the lake, and he was alone on land" (Mk 6:46-47).

Sometimes Jesus chose to end his day in prayer. Once, for example, after a long day of teaching the crowds and then providing food for them by a miracle, he left his inner circle and headed for a place in the mountains. What did Jesus do there? He spent time in communion with his Father. Perhaps Jesus realized that he needed the soul-rest that comes in communion with his Father *even more* than he needed physical rest in sleep. Do you and I realize this?

How might I follow Jesus in my evenings? What keeps *me* up late at night? Sometimes it is a mindless escape into less-than-stellar television programming. Sometimes a video game that captures me. Sometimes a snack that I really don't need. Sometimes a project I didn't finish during my daylight hours but am trying to make progress on—at maybe 20 percent efficiency. Or do I sometimes choose to stay up late, after others have retired to their beds, to enjoy those quieter, less-likely-to-be-interrupted moments and be attentive to the presence of the One who calls me his beloved, to listen for his voice and watch for his face? Jesus must have felt he would more likely find what he most needed that night in the presence of his Father than he would with his head on his pillow.

"One of those days Jesus went out to a mountainside to pray, and spent the night praying to God. When morning came, he called his disciples to him and chose twelve of them, whom he also designated apostles" (Lk 6:12-13).

According to Luke, Jesus left behind the community of followers, went out to a mountainside and spent an unhurried night in prayerful communion with the Father. He committed himself to this level of prayer on the night before he chose the Twelve out of the multitude of disciples who were already following him. These

twelve were to be his key leaders, and Jesus knew that he needed
the Father's perspective, the Father's wisdom, as he made his selec-
tions. Spirit-enabled to see each one through the Father's eyes,
Jesus then knew which ones to choose.

After an unhurried night of praying, listening to the Father,
sharing his own heart and perhaps praying for the larger group of
his followers, Jesus was able to see which men the Father was inviting into the inner circle. The Spirit guided Jesus in his leadership decisions, in this case decisions about which leaders to
select. In contrast, how many leadership decisions do I make based
on my initial reaction rather than on a more prayer-seasoned perspective? I am learning to seek God with diligence when I need to
make critical decisions like the selection of leaders. I no longer
presume that my first impulse is the best one.

How do you make the big decisions in your life? For example, if
you were assigned the task to choose twelve individuals to share
life with and to train to carry on your work after you leave, how
would you go about it? Would your immediate instinct be to first
spend many hours, even at the cost of sleep, to listen well for the
Father's guiding voice before you acted? Or would you first read
the résumés, check the references and conduct the interviews? And
while you're thinking about this, would you have picked the same
twelve Jesus did? I'm not sure I would have.

Jesus' choice of who would compose his core group was seasoned in his unhurried communion with his Father, informed by
divine wisdom rather than confined by conventional wisdom. Yet
much has been said about the twelve individuals Jesus chose.
Their résumés were not impressive or perhaps even relevant to
the position they sought. Yet, in the presence of his Father and
guided by the Holy Spirit, Jesus was able to see those twelve not
as they were then so much as who they would become as his followers over time.

How might I follow this pattern in Jesus' life? Perhaps I'd be intentional about making more time to be in God's presence before I make strategic decisions like the one Jesus made. And if Jesus himself invested an entire night in prayer before choosing his inner circle, how much more would I benefit from such an investment of time in prayer? The Father has an open door for you and me. He is available for our extensive and intensive communion with him whenever we face important decisions or difficult situations. Unfortunately—but not surprisingly—when I face key decisions in my own life and work, my own hurried, if not reactive, evaluation and my limited perspective often fail to be as wise or good as Jesus' was. Why? Perhaps because I fail to follow his mountaintop example. Unhurried time with the Father broadens our perspective and clarifies our vision. God enables us to see what we might look right past. So when Jesus made a choice seasoned in unhurried communion with his Father, that decision was enriched by divine wisdom and guidance.

When you imagine Jesus spending the night praying to God, do you picture him delivering a marathon monologue to the Father? Did his mouth grow dry and his mind grow numb from all the talk, all the arguments and counterarguments, the pros and cons for this person and that one? I don't think so. These extended times that Jesus set aside to be with the Father lead me to imagine a much more conversational kind of prayer between Jesus and the Father, including those precious moments of silence that are a sure sign of intimate friendship.

DISCERNING THE RHYTHM OF JESUS

As I wait and watch in the quiet this morning, I see the thinnest strip of light gray-blue along the Saddleback Ridge. A light, steady breeze cools my face. I feel God with me. Yet as I sit in this outward quiet, I feel inward noise arise. I feel my soul tempted by familiar anxiety and fear. In the quiet, I'm able to recognize that this worry and fear *never* come from the Lord: "Father, help me walk today in your grace and peace, with holy energy and creativity for the work you have for me to do today."

This experiment makes me feel the high resolve it took for Jesus to regularly withdraw from the many expectations and demands of the disciples and the crowds, his resolve to live unhurriedly in communion with the Father. If Jesus hadn't left the house in the predawn hours, he would certainly have been awakened and called on to serve. He wanted to engage his Father first. He wanted to hear the voice of the One who had already been saying, "You are my Son, whom I love; with you I am well pleased" (Mk 1:11). Who wouldn't want to start the day hearing that voice above all others?

Reviewing and reflecting on the pages of the Gospels, I find myself asking basic questions about Jesus' rhythm of prayer. What insights do we gain from the way Jesus prayed? What does Jesus show us about how to practice unhurried time with the Father?

When? Jesus often prayed at times when very little other activity would be going on, such as early in the morning or late at night. He didn't hesitate to rise before sunrise or stay up well after sunset, and we know that he even stayed up all night. Clearly, Jesus made a special effort to have regular uninterrupted time with his Father. It was a life-giving habit for him, but I don't believe the habit was easy for him. After all, he was as fully human as we are. He must have felt tired early in the morning or late at night just as we do. But Jesus so treasured communion alone with his Father that nothing else was more important to him.

How frequently? One text (Lk 5:16) reports that Jesus *often* went off on his own to pray like this. Solitary prayer was his regular habit.

Where? Jesus often went to remote locations when he prayed. He sought out places where he would be alone with God. He left a house and the village where he was staying to walk to a more deserted place. One Gospel passage called this *withdrawing*: Jesus got away from the many demands on him and his time in order to enjoy the Father's presence. It appears that Jesus enjoyed natural outdoor settings, like a mountainside, for times of personal prayer, yet he also encouraged his followers to go to their closet to pray in secret before the Father.

With whom? Sometimes Jesus prayed alone: he chose locations that provided solitude. Sometimes Jesus even sent the disciples away so that he could have time alone with God in prayer. And Jesus had times of prayer with his disciples as well. At more pivotal moments, like the transfiguration and Gethsemane, he prayed with Peter, James and John.

How long? The biblical texts don't say much here, but one text tells us that Jesus spent all night in prayer before selecting his disciples. Jesus probably did a great deal of praying during his forty days in the desert when his ministry began. Other biblical texts suggest that Jesus devoted significant amounts of time to prayer. Those reports that he withdrew to a lonely place, prayed and returned clearly imply a significant investment of time.

Yet these few lines about how Jesus prayed during his three years of public ministry have rarely been in focus for me. In all my years as a Christian, I have rarely, if ever, heard mention made of these vignettes from the life of Jesus or of his rich communion with the Father. Sermons I've heard about Jesus have tended to focus on his ministry activities; they have often overlooked the rich inner life that fueled all that Jesus actually said and did.

JESUS AND HIS FIRST FOLLOWERS

Let's look a little closer at Jesus' intentionality with his first followers. I think of a time when the demands of the crowd overwhelmed the disciples: "Then, because so many people were coming and going that they did not even have a chance to eat, he said to them, 'Come with me by yourselves to a quiet place and get some rest.' So they went away by themselves in a boat to a solitary place" (Mk 6:31-32).

Jesus invited his followers, in the midst of a busy time of ministering, to withdraw—as he often did—to a quiet, restful place where they could spend time in communion with the Father. Just as often as we need it, Jesus extends this same invitation to get away to a quiet, secluded place with him. Just as surely as God gives us ministry opportunities, he also gives us opportunities to rest with him and be restored. Are we open to both kinds of invitations? When we fail to open the Lord's invitations to rest, we behave as though God were a slave driver and we, the helpless slaves. But we are, first and foremost, God's beloved sons and daughters, invited to serve him and others in love, not out of any kind of obligation.

As Luke's story of Jesus continues, we find another time when he had been praying. This time, his disciples were witnesses: "One day Jesus was praying in a certain place. When he finished, one of his disciples said to him, 'Lord, teach us to pray, just as John taught his disciples'" (Lk 11:1). What finally compelled the disciples to consider following Jesus' way of praying was his *habit* of praying. They had witnessed this pattern in Jesus' life and could not ignore it. His communion with the Father kindled within them a desire for similar communion. Their request wasn't theoretical, but personal—and it underscores an important point. If we want to lead like Jesus, our own rhythm of prayer may be what provokes, inspires, even tantalizes others to seek our help and mentoring.

WHEN MINISTRY RUSHES US PAST JESUS

As Jesus and his disciples were on their way, he came to a village where a woman named Martha opened her home to him. She had a sister called Mary, who sat at the Lord's feet listening to what he said. But Martha was distracted by all the preparations that had to be made. She came to him and asked, "Lord, don't you care that my sister has left me to do the work by myself? Tell her to help me!"

"Martha, Martha," the Lord answered, "you are worried and upset about many things, but few things are needed—or indeed only one. Mary has chosen what is better, and it will not be taken away from her." (Lk 10:38-42)

Jesus visited his friends, Mary, Martha and Lazarus, in their home. In response to Martha's frantic and busy preparations, Jesus urged her to relax and simply be with him. E. Glenn Hinson offers this insight:

Jesus did not censure Martha's work, her ministry. Rather, he faulted her failure in her busyness to make the most of the present moment. Mary, the account says, "sat at the Lord's feet" and listened to what he was saying. But Martha was busying herself with a lot of ministry (*diakonia*). You can readily understand and may sympathize with the exasperation Martha felt as she saw her sister. "She [Martha] stopped and said, 'Sir, doesn't it bother you that my sister sits there on her can and leaves me to do all the work? Tell her to get up and help me'" (Luke 10:40, AP). Precisely how you may feel when you see people sitting around while you work![3]

Martha's worried words to Jesus exposed her hurried heart. Doing something good *for* him took precedence over listening to something good *from* him.

DID THEY KEEP FOLLOWING?

Did Jesus' first followers continue his priority of prayer in ministry after he ascended into heaven? One story that helps answer this question is found in Acts 6.

> So the Twelve gathered all the disciples together and said, "It
> would not be right for us to neglect the ministry of the word
> of God in order to wait on tables. Brothers and sisters, choose
> seven men from among you who are known to be full of the
> Spirit and wisdom. We will turn this responsibility over to
> them and will give our attention to prayer and the ministry of
> the word." (Acts 6:2-4)

These words, spoken by Jesus' Twelve, help me think about
what they had learned from him about spiritual leadership of God's
people. On what did Jesus want his leadership core to focus their
attention and activity? Critical and real needs. In this case, the
many widows could easily have taken up all of the disciples' time
and still not have had all their needs met. The women were hungry;
their needs were urgent. Certain widows were being helped and
others were not. Compassion demanded a response to this inequity.

I'm impressed with the disciples' twofold response. First, they
asked the community to choose godly, wise leaders from among
them to work on meeting this practical need. Second, they themselves continued to focus on "prayer and the ministry of the word."

In my own leadership places, how much time do I spend
"waiting on tables" and how much time do I spend in prayer and
Scripture? People will always have needs, and the community of
God's people must address these needs. We cannot say that we love
God and are walking in his ways yet ignore the needs of the people
among us. That said, there is a critical need for key leaders among
us who will give their full attention to God—to knowing him and
making him known. They must continue to cultivate a listening
heart in prayer. They must know what the Lord is saying to his
people in a particular place at a particular time. They must be prepared to speak on his behalf to the wider body of Christ. Since

none of us lives by bread alone (or by the work we do to produce and provide bread), we must have those church leaders who are always ready to provide us with the bread of life.

I'm not saying this is easy. I am very aware that the many urgencies of my life crowd out significant and extended times of prayer for the people of God, times of reflective study of Scripture and rich biblical instruction for God's people. So I ask the Father to give me courage to act on these truths from Acts 6 by entrusting some of the "waiting on tables" responsibilities to godly men and women in the community of believers.

Let me share one story of how this might look. Many years ago, I met a pastor of a small church (I'll call him Jim) who came to The Journey training. He was a very tired pastor, and was already thinking about leaving church ministry and teaching instead. (He had a Ph.D. in New Testament studies from a prestigious university, so a professorship wouldn't have been a difficult option for him to pursue.) As I listened to Jim describe his typical week as a pastor, I was overwhelmed just hearing about it. He was expected to be at every meeting held by any group in the church—board meetings, youth meetings, adult Bible studies, women's meetings, social events, you name it. His life was an unending series of meetings. There was no time in his schedule for anything like study, prayer or rest.

After that first retreat and hearing some insights about Jesus' pattern of withdrawal and engagement, Jim decided to take Thursday mornings to be alone with God in his office. During that time he would reflect on Scripture (on texts he would be preaching on in the next few weeks) and pray. He let the congregation know about his plan and asked that they not call or visit him on Thursday mornings. He also gave them the name and number of a person they could contact in case of emergency.

When Jim returned to the second Journey retreat, he was en-

couraged and energized. He shared that those weekly mornings
had been life-saving for him. He felt soul-nourished and encouraged
by those times of uninterrupted fellowship with the Father. One
unexpected fruit was that, according to the comments of his congregation, his weekly messages had dramatically improved. As
time went on, Jim continued to build into his schedule other patterns of withdrawal: he wanted to be with God in the midst of
faithful engagement in the work of ministry. Again, the congregation noticed and appreciated the fruit growing in his life as well
as the new ways he was shepherding them, so they welcomed his
new rhythms. A new rhythm may be exactly what you need. I know
that is a need for me, and I know the Lord will help.

Making Leadership Prayer a Priority

Some of us are paid in Christian leadership roles. Others volunteer
our time to serve. As a leader myself, I think about Jesus' rhythm of
ministry and prayer. What is inviting to me? What resistance rises
up within me? For example, to what degree do I see prayer as a
strategic activity of leaders in general and of my leadership responsibilities in particular? Am I tempted to see praying as something
others do for me and for my job? I'm a leader and those folks are
"pray-ers." I only need to look in the Bible. God's appointed leaders
are pray-ers. Wasn't Paul? How about Jesus? One of the single most
fruitful activities in which a leader can engage is praying—praying
for the people God has entrusted to our care.

As a paid Christian leader, I ask myself whether prayer is legitimate work during office hours or whether I should do it only "on
my own time." Do I see the office as the place where I do the important stuff, where I deal with paperwork, prepare messages, run
the institution, plan events, keep appointments, talk on the phone
and get things done? Is it at all possible that our office hours could
reflect the kind of time that the early church leadership spent to-

gether sharing in the Word, praying and enjoying fellowship (Acts 1–2)? And is it possible that I might do every task or conduct every meeting in a spirit of prayer? Are we living, as Paul implied, first and foremost as brothers in Christ and then fellow workers and fellow ministers (Col 4:7-11)? Does the way we spend our time together reflect these biblical priorities?

Frank Laubach, a missionary to the Philippines known for his *Letters by a Modern Mystic*, began to experiment with practicing God's presence when he first arrived on the mission field. In those early months, Laubach described himself as "a lonesome man in a strange land." He had a lot of time on his hands with which to give focused time to noticing God's presence and work. After a while, the demands of ministry began to increase, and Laubach was with people every moment of every waking day. In that context, he wrote:

> Either this new situation will crowd God out or I must take Him into it all. I must learn a continuous silent conversation of heart to heart with God while looking into other eyes and listening to other voices. If I decide to do this it is far more difficult than the thing I was doing before. Yet if this experiment is to have any value for busy people it must be worked under exactly these conditions of high pressure and throngs of people.[4]

What Frank Laubach described is the real world where we seek to cultivate moment-to-moment communion with God. Few of us are monks living in seclusion. Most of us live in a world of noise, demands and expectations. We can learn to make space for God as we arrive at the office, a ministry leadership meeting, a neighborhood block party—wherever. We are invited to live in such a hurried world somehow unhurried in our walk and work with God.

Let me end this chapter with a prayer: *Jesus, I long to live in loving communion with the Father like you did in your earthly life and as you do now. Slow me down from all my self-defined God projects that keep me from listening well to the voice of the One who says both, "I love you" and "I send you." Amen.*

UNHURRIED TIME

1. What is God doing to cultivate in me a greater awareness of him in my own life and in my community of faith?

2. In what ways does attending to the many needs and expectations of people around us crowd out time spent in prayer and in Scripture?

3. When you hear the word *prayer*, do you feel welcomed in God's presence or guilty for lack of personal faithfulness to such a practice? How might you enter into prayer as a relationship with One who loves and enjoys you without measure?

7

REST

The Rhythm of Creation

I struggle with rest. I often find restlessness rising up within me uninvited and unexpected. At such times, words from Hebrews 4 have been an oasis for me: "There remains, then, a Sabbath-rest for the people of God; for anyone who enters God's rest also rests from their works, just as God did from his. Let us, therefore, make every effort to enter that rest, so that no one will perish by following their example of disobedience" (Heb 4:9-11). Read those words again. Did you hear them? Do you believe them? Do I? Do we really believe that God has a "Sabbath-rest" for us—and, if we do, what is that rest all about?

God knows the value of rest. He himself rested, and he has designed us to rest, and to rest regularly—as in every seven days. Yet many believers today have not received the gift or entered into the rhythm of that rest. God nevertheless has that gift ready for his people's taking. In our North American context, we have to release habits of drivenness, anxiety and workaholism if we are to receive the gift of rest. We also need to turn to God and learn rest from the One who rested from his work of creation.

Some believers, however, will read "enter that rest" as an end-of-life goal rather than a here-and-now reality. That idea is certainly present in the context of Hebrews, but that understanding can lead to a "work now, rest later" scenario. Others say, "I'd rather burn out than rust out for God." By this, they seem to mean that they would rather work for the Lord until they are totally out of gas than fail to work for him at all. I understand that sentiment, but, frankly, I would rather do neither. I long to live beneath the easy and well-fitting yoke of Jesus, a yoke that isn't burdensome or exhausting.

Sabbath is no afterthought; rather, Sabbath rest is primary, and our good work grows out of our rest. That is not how we think in twenty-first-century Western culture. We see work as primary and rest coming afterward. Eugene Peterson, pastor and translator of *The Message* version of the Bible, reminds us otherwise:

> The Hebrew evening/morning sequence conditions us to the rhythms of grace. We go to sleep, and God begins his work. As we sleep he develops his covenant. We wake and are called out to participate in God's creative action. We respond in faith, in work. But always grace is previous. Grace is primary. We wake into a world we didn't make, into a salvation we didn't earn. Evening: God begins, without our help, his creative day. Morning: God calls us to enjoy and share and develop the work he initiated. Creation and covenant are sheer grace and there to greet us every morning.[1]

The Hebrew mindset saw the day beginning with rest, not with work. In the West, our day begins at sunrise and, basically, with work. This sequence, as Peterson points out, is telling. We tend to see rest as the place we fall into after we've worn ourselves out with work. But what if our best work *begins* from a place of rest? What if rest takes first priority rather than last?

The primacy of rest, or Sabbath, is also illustrated in the story of creation. For the first few days, God created the heavens and the earth, separating light from darkness, waters from land, and sky from ground. He created sun, moon and stars and then a rich variety of plants and animals to populate the earth and oceans. Not until the sixth day did God create humankind, charging them to be fruitful, to multiply and to take care of the world he created. But before human beings could begin to do that, they were to observe the seventh day as Sabbath. There's no evidence that they had done anything to subdue the earth through their labor yet. Instead, they begin their lives with rest, not work.

Abraham Heschel, one of the leading Jewish theologians of the twentieth century, suggests that "the Sabbath is a day for the sake of life. Man is not a beast of burden, and the Sabbath is not for the purpose of enhancing the efficiency of his work. 'Last in creation, first in intention,' the Sabbath is 'the end of the creation of heaven and earth.'"[2] In Hebrews 4, God invites us to "make every effort to enter that rest." I can't help but think that this sounds like a contradiction. It seems either I "make every effort" *or* I "enter . . . rest," yet we're told to make every effort to enter the rest God has for us. As each one of us knows, living a truly restful life isn't as easy as it may sound. We have a lot of restlessness in us. And since you and I live in a culture that tends to measure people by what they *do*, the prospect of resting, of doing nothing for a season, can feel like volunteering for a loss of identity. Who am I if I'm not producing something, achieving something, accomplishing something?[3]

This need to produce or do is often as present in the church as it is in the world. I work with pastors and other Christian leaders, and many of them are among the very driven. We can be frantic in our work *for* God. But what if all the work I'm doing *for* him isn't always work that he has given me to do? What if I'm making the yoke of service heavier than he means it to be? He calls his yoke easy and his burden light (see Mt 11:29-30). My failure to live and work restfully makes my yoke of service harder and heavier than it should be.

GOD'S RESTLESS PEOPLE

Consider what we can learn from the bad example of the Israelites in Exodus 17:1-7. The Israelites have been wandering in the wilderness awhile when they come to a place where there is nothing to drink. They get thirsty, they complain and they demand that Moses give them water. They complain that God isn't taking care of them. So God tells Moses to strike the rock with his staff as the elders and the people watch. After all, the Lord had promised that his presence would be with Moses and the Israelites, so here he provides them with water. Moses, however, calls the place *Massah* ("testing") and *Meribah* ("quarrelling") because of the Israelites' behavior and attitude.

The Israelites failed to enter into God's rest because they chose to test God instead of trust him. They quarreled with God instead of following him. And these are the same reasons you and I fail to enter his rest today. We test God when we trust in our own work more than we trust in his; we quarrel with God when we struggle and strive with him instead of resting and trusting.

UNHURRY ROOTED IN CREATION

The Sabbath is God's antidote for our hurried, harried pace of life, and gives us the unhurried one-in-seven rhythm woven into the very fabric of creation. That seventh day is a space for us to enter into needed recovery (and perhaps go through the inevitable withdrawals) from the hurry, drivenness and workaholism that plague so many of our lives, families, communities and organizations. On the Sabbath, hurry becomes a vice, the exact opposite of our workaday world's way of making it a virtue. The Sabbath gives us a holy rhythm designed to slow us so that we might better love God and love others.

Spiritual director and psychiatrist Gerald May describes the Sabbath as a "day of spaciousness in form, time, and soul." He continues: "Now, religious Sabbath is apt to feel like restriction rather than freedom, confinement rather than space. Instead of freedom from having to work, Sabbath came to mean not being *allowed* to work."[4] Ironically, a generation ago, experts predicted that at this point in time we would be living in an era of unprecedented leisure thanks to labor-saving technologies that were beginning to proliferate then. They envisioned a future (our present) in which tasks that took up much of our lives would take much less time or even be done without much direct human effort at all.

But the reality is that today, we as a culture feel more hurried and less relaxed than perhaps we've ever felt. Technology has indeed enabled us to do certain kinds of work in less time. We have not, however, taken advantage of this gift to make more space for Sabbath leisure. Most of us have instead chosen to do even more work, using more time to make more money and purchase more things that won't really satisfy us. We have chosen—and continue to choose—more hurry instead of more leisure. We've tended to choose money over time. *That* is, in fact, the problem of modern life that no one could foresee.

So, in light of both this ongoing choice of busyness over rest and the Hebrews invitation to "enter his rest," perhaps the greatest leadership challenge any of us faces is ordering our days rightly, giving appropriate priority to our spiritual life. But the state of our spiritual life is one aspect of our life that others rarely seem to ask about. With that topic often ignored in everyday conversation, the matter seems nonurgent, and we forget just how important the pace of our life is.

Allen Johnson, professor emeritus of anthropology at UCLA, makes this important and quite sobering point:

> As a result of producing and consuming more, we are experiencing an increasing scarcity of time. This works in the

following way. Increasing efficiency in production means that each individual must produce more goods per hour; increasing productivity means . . . that to keep the system going we must consume more goods. Free time gets converted into consumption time because time spent neither producing nor consuming comes increasingly to be viewed as wasted. . . . The increase in the value of time (its increasing scarcity) is felt subjectively as an increase in tempo or pace. We are always in danger of being slow on the production line or late to work; and in our leisure we are always in danger of wasting time.[5]

We are a culture that measures value in terms of production or consumption. If the Sabbath is a day set aside each week to cease both of these activities, it's easy to see why our contemporary culture views it as a waste of a day.

The Doorway to the Sabbath

At the heart of understanding the value of the Sabbath is simple trust. The writer of Hebrews says that those who enter God's rest are the ones who "share the faith of those who obeyed" (4:2). In other words, the doorway into experiencing God's rest in our lives is faith. It takes trust in God's faithfulness to choose to stop our work. When we choose soul rest, we are putting our trust in God's work, not our own, and we then experience the gift of Sabbath. Author and pastor Marc Buchanan makes this connection when he says, "Sabbath [is about trust]. Sabbath is turning over to God all those things—our money, our work, our status, our reputations, our plans, our projects—that we're otherwise tempted to hold tight in our own closed fists, hold on to for dear life."[6]

The gift of a Sabbath day—a day measured not by productivity but by relationship and worship—helps us remember and trust that life is given, not earned. But we live in a culture that expects us to earn everything we have. In *Spiritual Direction*, Henri Nouwen gets more specific, suggesting that we live in a culture where our identity is based on how well we do, how much we do, how much we possess and what others say about us.[7] When these factors are the source of our identity, it's not hard to understand why we are hurrying through life. The thinking—however conscious or unconscious—goes like this: *If I do more, I am more. If I have more, I am more. If more people like and recognize me more, I'm more valuable.* This idea is subtle, and insidious in its undermining of the Sabbath. What happens to our sense of identity if we stop our activity to observe the Sabbath day? If I am what I do, who am I on a Sabbath day when I do nothing productive?

We err when we try to *establish* our identity through our work rather than realizing that our identity is shaped and strengthened in the place of Sabbath rest and then *expressed* in our work. We have it backward, and our language reveals that fact. I know you've heard people say—and maybe you've said it yourself—"I'm going to lose myself in my work." These people are saying more than they realize! And their statement suggests we need to recover our lives in Sabbath places with Jesus.

During a ministry sabbatical year, I wrestled deeply with the question "Who am I if I'm not counseling and teaching others, if I don't have a ministry position or if I have nothing happening in my life that might impress others?" The deep anxieties that arose in me were evidence of where my trust—my faith—was actually rooted: I had more confidence in my own work to give me value than I had in God's work on the cross.

During that year, I read Tilden Edwards's book *Sabbath Time.* I needed his insights about these dynamics within me that were so frustrating and difficult to understand. Edwards, a prolific author and wise spiritual director, suggests the following:

An understanding and living of Sabbath time can help support a sane and holy rhythm of life for us. With it, we are given an alternative to the culture's growing movement between driven achievement and narrow escape time. Instead of this deadly rhythm, we can find ourselves in the authentic classical Christian rhythm of ministry and Sabbath. This rhythm intrinsically can witness to and teach much about the Christian way.[8]

Edwards suggests two very different rhythms of life: first, an unhealthy cycle of driven achievement and narrow escape time, and second, the healthy rhythm of ministry/work and Sabbath.

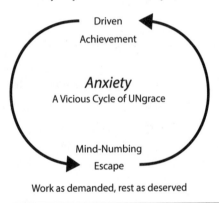

Figure 7.1

The cultural cycle of drivenness and escape is a counterfeit of the more biblical rhythm of work and Sabbath. At the heart of the culture's cycle is anxiety, and anxiety drives us to do, do and then do some more. Over time, anxiety exhausts us until we want to escape to anywhere that we won't have to *do* anything. In this cycle, we experience work as demanded of us by others (or even by ourselves) and rest as deserved. There is very little grace in this view of work and rest.

Furthermore, hurry makes life feel like an unending series of "have tos"—life "have tos," family "have tos," work "have tos" and so on. On a Sabbath day, however, we Christians may, in a radical and countercultural way, step away from this "have to" orientation and enter into a holy "want to" place. There, we can let that hurried, pressured orientation to life and ministry lift, and get in touch with the God-given "want tos" that can really move us in living his life and engaging his work. When the "have tos" stop swirling, the "want tos" can float back to the surface of our heart and the forefront of our mind. Then we can remember *why* we are doing some of the whats we are doing. This remembering gives us purpose and is one reason why we need the rhythm of Sabbath in our workweek.

A biblical illustration of this truth is found in Deuteronomy 5, where Moses recounts the Ten Commandments. There, Moses reminds the people that they were slaves in Egypt, and the implication is that, as slaves of demanding taskmasters, they were not *free* to observe the Sabbath (Deut 6:12-15). When we fail to make space for Sabbath rest in our schedules, we are behaving as though we are slaves too. God never meant Sabbath to be an enslaving, "you can't" day as much as a freeing, "you don't have to" day. We act as though we have no freedom to choose to make regular space for rest in our life and work.

REMEMBERING HOLY DESIRE

This idea of freedom reminds me of my decision to pursue ministry as my life's vocation. Few who engage in ministry, either as a vocation or as a volunteer, do so because of obligation or compulsion. Instead, most have a deep longing to share the life of God they have come to know and appreciate.

When I decided I wanted to be a pastor, no one had put me in a headlock. I wasn't compelled by guilt or shame to make that decision. I just wanted others to know the transformation of life that I was experiencing. I *wanted* to serve God's purposes in the lives of other people. I wasn't excited about making a mark on the ministry landscape. Instead, I was very excited about others meeting and coming to know Christ in a deeper and deeper way. But sometimes the growing list of paid ministry's "need tos" and "have tos" bury that original desire. In fact, the longer I was in church ministry, and the longer my to-do list became, the taller my inbox pile grew and the fuller my calendar became, the more I felt overwhelmed by "have-to-itis." My holy desire became smothered underneath it all. Unhurried time enables the reality of holy desire to return to the surface and move me once again to holy action.

Simply put, hurry can cause us to forget our sense of God-given purpose.

Tilden Edwards describes how this particular individualized way of life can then cause us to "collapse into some form of oblivion: sleep, drink, drugs, any kind of television, or whatever else might numb our self-production for a while."[9] I confess: I do have a few places I'm tempted to go when I want to numb out. The first is television, where wonderful educational programs, engaging dramas and exciting sports events are available to me. These shows can be energizing, fun and wonderful to share with others. But sometimes the way I watch television is much more numbing. With a somewhat glassy stare, I sit with a remote in my hand and cycle through all the available channels. I don't sit down to be inspired, instructed or stirred. If I'm honest with myself, I will admit that I am looking to be numbed. And being numb is not the same as resting in the Lord. I can't remember getting up after watching an hour or two of television thinking, *Wow! I've never felt more alive!* Usually, I feel more tired and mildly depressed.[10]

Another misguided way I—and others—seek rest is comfort eating. When I'm making my way to the pantry or the refrigerator at 11:00 p.m., it's not because I need some sustenance for the hours of hard work that lie ahead of me. I do not work the night shift in my ministry! Even though satisfying a craving for something sweet or crunchy or salty or fatty has yet to bring rest to my soul, I often end up going there anyway.

The biblical and far more life-giving rhythm of Sabbath and ministry/work is illustrated in figure 7.2.

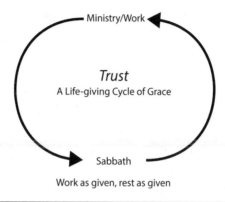

Figure 7.2

As figure 7.2 shows, at the heart of this rhythm is trust. In trust, we receive grace as the living center, meaning we recognize that work is not demanded but given, and rest is not deserved but also given. Rest and work are both gifts from God. Getting up earlier and staying up later to get more and more done is empty when we realize that God *gives* rest to the ones he loves (Ps 127:2). We are God's creative work in Christ, meant to do the good work that he prepared ahead for us to engage in (Eph 2:10). But when we live according to the cultural pattern, our version of rest often ends up more like anesthesia than refreshment.

I experienced this holy rhythm firsthand when I spent a month in the midst of my one-year sabbatical at the Pecos Benedictine Abbey in New Mexico for training in the art of spiritual direction. It was my first personal exposure to the Benedictine rhythm of life, work and prayer. I found that there was enough time in the day for everything that needed to be done. There was no sense of hurry. One reason is—as Joan Chittister, a Benedictine writer and lecturer, points out—that "leisure . . . is an essential part of Benedictine spirituality. It is not laziness and it is not selfishness. It has something to do with depth and breadth, length and quality of life."[11] I am coming to realize that there is holy leisure and there is unholy leisure.

How do we discern the difference between holy and unholy leisure? Holy leisure is life-giving; unholy leisure is life-draining. But activities don't always fit neatly into these categories. I might, for instance, play a video game with one of my sons, and we might find it energizing and fun. But I might play that same video game for hours on end, in isolation, and afterward feel numb and empty inside. I might take a walk along an ocean bluff with my wife and feel invigorated by the gift of companionship and natural beauty, or I might head for the ocean to escape the good work God has prepared for me to do on a particular day. Whether an activity makes for holy or unholy leisure often has more to do with what's going on inside of me than what the particular activity is.

As I mentioned, I've learned from my Benedictine brothers and sisters that their rhythm of life provides enough time for a balance of what is good—work and prayer, reflection and study, solitude and community. They helped me realize that I hurry, in part, because I labor under the false belief that I don't have enough time for what is good and necessary for me. Somehow I behave as though Jesus was wrong when he said that his yoke is well-fitting and his burden is light (Mt 11:30). Holy leisure is a way of recognizing that everything God has invited me to do can be done without anxious hurry. The rule of Benedict helps create a rhythm that honors this wisdom. That's not to say that I won't have very full days—and nights—along the way. But may such times remain seasons and not become my constant pace. I don't want to just be skimming across the surface of my life.

Joan Chittister goes on to say this:

Leisure has two dimensions, play and rest. The Benedictine
Rule does not talk about play because play was built right into
sixth-century life by the church calendar. One of the functions
of holy days and festivals, most of which started in churches
and religious communities, was to provide both the privileged
and the peasants of the society with space and time for
common enjoyment. On Church feasts commoners could not
be required to work. Play was the Church's gift to the working
class in a day before labor unions and industrialization.[12]

Play was so natural for me as a child and a youth, but that has
faded in my adult life. I don't find myself as playful now as I was
even as a young adult. Recently, my family and I spent the evening
in our living room playing Catch Phrase. At first, I could feel resistance rising: "I really have important things I should be doing. I
feel like being alone. And I'm not really a game player."

But in a moment of God-given awakening, I realized how thin
and silly those excuses were. It was evening. At that moment, what
was more important than unhurried time spent enjoying my bride
and my three teenaged sons? Was anything better waiting for me in
the cave that is my home office? No! And why couldn't I be a little
more playful with my family? We ended up laughing and talking
together for a couple of hours. When it was over I could tell that it
had been life-giving for each one of us. I could take away a lesson
from my Benedictine friends. Clearly, times like this form a life-
sustaining trellis on which good things can grow.

Also addressing the importance of play, writer Stuart Brown lists
some properties of play, including that it's "apparently purposeless
(done for its own sake)" and involves "freedom from time" and
"diminished consciousness of self."[13] Unlike work that results in a
mortgage payment or a cleaner house, real play is an activity that

has no obviously profitable purpose. Play is not for the purpose of accomplishing something. In fact, it is the opposite: play pushes the pause button on our tendency toward—or, for some, our habit of—unceasing productivity.

THE TIME FOR SABBATH REST

Returning to Hebrews 4:7, we're reminded through David that the Lord set a certain day—calling it "Today"—for his people to hear his voice with receptive, responsive hearts. "Today" is the day we enter into God's gift of Sabbath, his gift of rest. Unfortunately, when it comes to rest, we tend to turn "Today" into "Someday." Someday I'll live a more restful life. *When I get out of college and start my career . . . When I get married and start a family . . . When I get established in my life and job . . . When I retire . . . When I die?* When will we "enter his rest"? We default to that out-of-reach "Someday" whenever we offer up our "not yet" excuses. Sometimes it's a seasonal "not yet": "I just can't afford the time right now"; or an emotional "not yet": "Rest is a luxury I just can't afford"; or, finally, a social "not yet": "No one else is doing it!"

Why do you and I postpone God's gift of rest? Why do we procrastinate? I often fail to enjoy the gift of God's rest because I'm not willing to open my hands to receive it. In his book *Sabbath*, Wayne Muller reminds us that "Sabbath requires surrender. If we only stop when we are finished with all our work, we will never stop—because our work is never completely done. . . . If we refuse rest until we are finished, we will never rest until we die. Sabbath dissolves the artificial urgency of our days, because it liberates us from the need to be finished."[14] Sabbath can be a weekly reminder that our work is not sovereign, but God is. Our allegiance is first to God, not to our to-do list or appointment calendar. Today is the day to enter into a weekly rhythm of ceasing my work one day in seven. Here I more deeply remember that God's work always precedes mine.

Another reason I don't enter today into God-given rest is that I am overtired. It sounds silly, but Thomas Merton says as much:

> There are times, then, when in order to keep ourselves in existence at all we simply have to sit back for a while and do nothing. And for a man who has let himself be drawn completely out of himself by his activity, nothing is more difficult than to sit still and rest, doing nothing at all. The very act of resting is the hardest and most courageous act he can perform: and often it is quite beyond his power.[15]

Entering today into the rhythm of Sabbath spaces and times enables me to remember how special I am to the Father. A large part of my ministry these days is providing days of intentional solitude and silence for Christian leaders and people working for various ministries. I can't count how many times I've had a capable, high-energy leader come to such a day, often for the first time, and express deep anxiety and resistance to spending a number of hours "doing nothing" other than staying in God's presence. Taking this step really does require courage and faith, but what we find when we take it is that God is present, God is at work and God is involved in our lives.

God provided generous Sabbath space in the rhythm of Israel's life. We've already talked about the weekly day of rest he gave in the Sabbath, but in addition to those weekly places of rest, God gave a number of other spaces in their calendar. For example, the monthly New Moon festival was a Sabbath-like day on which no work was done.[16] So to the weekly Sabbath we can add the monthly New Moon festival (which might overlap two or three times a year). There were also the three major festivals of Passover ("unleavened bread"), Pentecost ("weeks") and Tabernacles ("ingathering"). These three feasts were pilgrimage events that could involve many days of travel to and from Jerusalem, and the first and last days of those weeks were Sabbath-like days on which no typical work was done (Lev 23:7-8). The Lord reiterates, in the context of these feasts, that his people must "rest, even during the plowing season and harvest" (Ex 34:21). If you add to this the command to let the land rest one year in seven when it was not to be planted, pruned or harvested (Lev 25:2-6) and the Jubilee Year (one in fifty), which was another Sabbath year for the land (Lev 25:8-12), there is a surprising amount of nonwork space God builds into the weekly, monthly, annual and lifetime rhythms of his people. If God provided that much space for his people to be together in his presence, how might we wish to open up at least a little more space in our own lives?

Unhurried Time

1. In what ways is God inviting you to open up even a little more Sabbath rest space in your life, your family and your work rhythms?

2. What arguments arise in the back of your mind that prevent you from "making every effort to enter his rest"? What answers would you like to give to these arguments?

3. When do you have times that aren't measured by what you produce, but instead by Sabbath values of relaxation, worship, love and even play?

SUFFERING

Unexpected Unhurrying

A few years ago, my wife suffered through what we came to call the "summer of pain." One day Gem was leaning over to make a bed, and a few weeks later she crumpled onto that bed in overwhelming sciatica pain. Watching someone you love endure great pain—physical or otherwise—is its own kind of suffering.

I remember taking her to almost daily chiropractic appointments (we were trying to avoid the uncertainty of surgery). I remember having to creep along with her as each step sent shooting pain down her leg. Our lives slowed down to a snail's pace because Gem couldn't move any faster, when she could move at all. We were living our lives at the unhurried—unable to hurry!—pace of pain.

Sometimes Gem would be awake in the middle of the night because she was between pain pills. I would walk back and forth at the foot of our bed praying psalms aloud, if only to try to distract her from how much her lower back was hurting. Sometimes it helped. Sometimes it didn't.

Around that time, I received a copy of the classic book by J. B. Phillips, *Your God Is Too Small*. One day while I waited for Gem's daily therapy, I read this in the introduction (and forgive

the male-focused language that reflects the times in which this
was written):

> It is obviously impossible for an adult to worship the con-
> ception of God that exists in the mind of a child of Sunday-
> school age, unless he is prepared to deny his own experience
> of life. If, by a great effort of will, he does do this he will
> always be secretly afraid lest some new truth may expose the
> juvenility of his faith. And it will always be by such an effort
> that he either worships or serves a God who is really too
> small to command his adult loyalty and cooperation.[1]

Gem's pain and my powerlessness exposed my own immature,
childish images of God. The pain in Gem's body drove me to
wonder aloud about God's actual care and his presence with us. I
felt his apparent absence more often than his obvious presence. I
wondered during the wrestlings of that season, *How long, O Lord?
How long does Gem have to hurt? How long until you bring comfort
and relief?*

After a few months of this, Gem's pain began to subside, and she
began to recover strength and freedom of movement. As hard as
that season was and as much as our trust was stretched, our faith
didn't reach a breaking point. But in that time of her intense suffering, we didn't care much about a biblical explanation of what
was happening and why. The pace of pain became, for us, the pace
of God's love and grace. We discovered that what we wanted most
was to know that God was with us.[2] And isn't that what all of us
need to know during the hardships, the challenges and the suf-
ferings of our lives?

God's Fierce Mercy

Let me share a little of our young married story. A few years into
our marriage, I came up against a place of suffering that was, in

many ways, of my own making. It was a season of burnout. I was overly busy and overworked. I came to recognize, though, that it was a severe form of God's many-faceted mercy that drove me to see my deep need for him. It was a deeply painful place, but God used it to take me to a much better place.

I know from my own wrestling with workaholism and from my work with others who seek to recover from this addictive dynamic that—and this is a painful realization—we have pursued work for God in order to escape the face of God. We have often felt justified in our out-of-balance life because we were doing the *work of God*. We don't have to be paid ministers to experience this. How can anyone argue with "I'm doing more work for God! Are you going to tell me to do less work for God?" Now my response would be "Are you sure it's the work of God? When did God tell you to do it? If you're carrying a yoke that's too heavy for you, are you telling Jesus he's wrong when he describes his own yoke as well-fitting and restful?" Again, I think sometimes pruning is the experience of God taking away from us something we thought was very fruitful but was in fact keeping us from being as fruitful as we could be.

Thanks to God's provision of a few key mentors at this time in my life, my wife and I both experienced a year of great renewal and spiritual encouragement—a year of God's favor. (I described this year in chapter two.) In that very same year, Gem received the news that her father's cancer had returned. He had fought a battle with cancer for decades. Now he was in his seventies, and cancer had returned with a vengeance. Over the course of that year, Gem and I watched this vital, energetic man be diminished week by week until there was hardly anything left of him. Perhaps you have walked through something like that with a loved one and know the pain of witnessing the suffering of a person you care about. We were both in our twenties, and this was our first experience with the death of someone close to us. The death of Gem's father made for a tough season of life for us. But there's no suffering harder than the one each of us may be facing now. Your suffering always feels the hardest because it's yours, right?

A year later, Gem discovered she was pregnant in the same moment she realized she was miscarrying. This was her second miscarriage, the first coming five years earlier. At that time, we were serving in a large Southern California church as pastors to college students. As we dealt with the pain and disappointment of our own miscarriages, we found ourselves in the position of counseling and caring for young women who were surprised to find themselves pregnant. They didn't want to be a parent; we did. Why wasn't God allowing us to receive the very gift that these young women didn't yet want?

A year later, Gem was pregnant a third time, and we learned early on that she faced a challenging pregnancy once again. When she experienced bleeding in the first trimester, the doctor did some testing and told us that Gem had a fibroid growing in the wall of her uterus—and it was growing faster than the baby was. Fearing a second- or third-trimester miscarriage, the doctor put Gem on bed rest for the majority of the pregnancy. We asked everyone we could think of to pray that the baby might outgrow the fibroid and come to full term. At the end of that hard, uncertain, touch-and-go season, we celebrated the arrival of our firstborn son: Sean came into the world after a long labor and finally a C-section. Six months later, a fibroid that had been nearly the size of a twin was removed. A hard but happy ending. (By the way, our prayer that Sean would outgrow the fibroid may not have been the smartest way to put our request. Sean has ended up being at the 99th percentile of growth his entire life, being six-foot-five now as a young adult!)

At about the time Sean was six months old and Gem was preparing to have fibroid surgery, I was invited into the senior pastor's office of the church where I had served for the first eight years of our married life. Money had been tight at the church, and I was told that there weren't funds for my position and I was being laid off. I had never seen anything like this happen in a church. In about a month, I would be without a job. Gem and I had recently purchased a home in the area. We were new parents. And we would very soon be without any visible means of support.

The loss of that ministry position raised many questions in me: *Who am I if I am not Pastor Alan? Who am I if I am not serving in a ministry role at a local church, if I am not doing what I have been doing my whole adult life until now? What value do I have if I'm not being paid to do this kind of work?* It took six months, but God provided us with a position in a smaller church, and we were blessed to lead a similar ministry to college students and young adults. But because the church was more than an hour from the one from which I had been released, we had to put our home up for sale. The market was down, and there weren't many bites.

A few months later, a little event called the Northridge earthquake hit. Our home was just over the hill in Simi Valley. The short version of the story is that our house experienced some damage—and no one was buying houses for months after that event! We couldn't afford a house payment in Simi and a rental payment elsewhere. There were no other options available to us than to give the house back to the bank, along with almost nine years of savings. Our possessions were reduced to what would fill a small moving truck.

A crisis a year. The death of a parent. The death of an unborn child. Fear of death during another pregnancy. Death of a ministry. A financial death. We struggled hard to have our eyes open to see the resurrections in the midst of those deaths.

Waiting

In that crisis-a-year season, we felt like we visited a lot of waiting rooms. Now, you might not think of waiting as suffering (though I suppose it depends some on what you are waiting for and for how long). Waiting isn't a sharp, crisis pain; instead, it is more of a dull, chronic ache that makes one wonder if it will ever go away. I find waiting, like patience, to be a great challenge. The older English word for *patience* was *long-suffering*. Patient waiting involves enduring discomfort—or worse—longer than we'd like.

In his commentary on "the dark night," John of the Cross used the image of a model sitting still before a master painter. He wrote, "If a model for the painting or retouching of a portrait should move because of a desire to do something, the artist would be unable to finish and the work would be spoiled."[3] I'm tempted to do something—*anything*—when I'm in one of life's waiting places. But maybe God has placed me there to be still and to wait on the creative work he is doing. That being the case, I must sit still so that the master painter can paint what he wishes. If I keep getting up to see what he is doing, I will make it hard for him to create the beauty he wants to create, if not spoil his work completely.

Paul's experience with the thorn in his side is another example of waiting. In 2 Corinthians 12, Paul said God had given him "surpassingly great revelations" (v. 7) that could have tempted him to self-importance or conceit, but "to keep me from becoming conceited, I was given a thorn in my flesh, a messenger of Satan." *Given?* A thorn in the flesh sure doesn't sound like a gift to me! "Three times I pleaded with the Lord to take it away from me" (v. 8). Wouldn't you ask? I know I would—and have! I'm sure Paul used all the appropriate words, offering his request in Jesus' name and all, but God's answer to that request was . . . an invitation to wait. Essentially God said, "No. I'm not removing the thorn. I have something better for you." I wonder if Paul appreciated the betterness of God's plan in that moment! How thrilled could he be in the moment when God was saying, "I'm going to give you my grace, and my grace is enough for you. After all, if I answered your request and took away the thorn, you would miss out on my plans for you. So I'm going to give you grace, enough grace, and keep the thorn in place, because my power is made perfect in weakness."

Does our theology of spiritual growth and leadership development include weakness that opens up space in our life for God's power? Or do we assume that human strength and wholeness are key to effective, fruitful leadership? I don't hear a lot of discussion about leadership in terms of *feeling* weak and *being* strong, like the model God outlined for Paul. Paul put it this way: "When I am weak, then I am strong" (v. 10). At one time, I assumed this sentence referred to a sequence of events: I would feel weak for a little while, and then I'd feel strong. I don't think that way anymore. I believe that sentence is describing something concurrent. *When* and *then* are happening in the same moment: grace makes me strong in the very moment I am feeling weak.

DRYNESS

Just as God's grace helps us through seasons of waiting, God also helps us through times of dryness. In those seasons of crisis, I remember many moments of deep dryness. When I talk about dryness, I'm not talking about the kind of dry that comes if we decide not to seek God, if we choose not to abide in him, if we elect to let busyness prevent us from the kind of communion that fills the cup of our lives. If we make these choices, we experience dryness, but it's a dryness that has a discernible cause. It's a dryness we can do something about. The dryness that I'm describing is an unexplained dryness. We are seeking God. We are entering into the kinds of practices that once opened us to God's refreshment, but we are finding ourselves not at an oasis but in a wilderness. No matter how hard we seek, we find ourselves still thirsting. I wonder if this was in David's heart when he prayed, "You, God, are my God, earnestly I seek you; I thirst for you, my whole being longs for you, in a dry and parched land where there is no water" (Ps 63:1).

I believe that there is a point in our spiritual journey when the Spirit will lead us into the desert just as he did Jesus. We hear the Spirit calling to us in the restlessness and weariness of our own heart. The first time the Spirit speaks to us in such a way, though, we don't recognize that the voice is his. We assume we're just not doing enough to be healthy and strong in soul, so we renew our religious efforts. I've seen that when we're in the dry places, God enables our longings for him to be deepened. And God has helped me see that if our longings for him were always easily fulfilled, they might not have the opportunity to become more deeply rooted. In other words, when we live with unfilled longings for a while, if we feel a thirst that is not quickly quenched, and if we resist the urge to escape into empty activities and false promises of refreshment or fullness, our longings are deepened and perhaps even strengthened.

I think of Paul's words:

We were under great pressure, far beyond our ability to endure, so that we despaired of life itself. Indeed, we felt we had received the sentence of death. But this happened that we might not rely on ourselves but on God, who raises the dead. (2 Cor 1:8-9)

Some commentators suggest that Paul's troubles here involved human opposition. Others think he faced a life-threatening illness. I haven't experienced a whole lot of either of these, but am I wrong to apply this verse to my own feelings of anxiety that often seem beyond my ability to endure? I'm sure that the pressure I feel is nowhere near what Paul felt, but it is very real pressure that can seem "beyond my ability to endure." I often, for instance, struggle to stand strong in the work God has given me in Jesus: He has called me to proclaim the goodness of an unhurried way. This message is a word of grace that so many of my brothers and sisters, trapped in a driven and draining way of life, so need to hear. No wonder I feel a kind of evil opposition to this work, and that opposition is a discouraging pressure that often feels beyond my endurance.

Why would God allow me to face extended seasons of pressure that feels far beyond my ability to endure? What might be his purpose? Paul shared that his own experience was about learning, together with his ministry colleagues, not to rely on himself but rather on the God who can raise the dead. The greater the challenge and the more deeply felt the overwhelming pressure, the greater can be my awareness that anything of eternal significance has nothing to do with me, myself or I. May I, like Paul, let God use every dry season of life—every season I spend in the wilderness— to learn to rely more on him.

The literal wilderness was, in fact, a classroom for the people of Israel: the dry, barren landscape was an important and difficult place of formation for them. They spent a lot of time there; the wilderness became much too familiar. Yet for generations afterward, Israel was urged to "remember how the LORD your God led you all the way in the wilderness these forty years, to humble and test you in order to know what was in your heart, whether or not you would keep his commands" (Deut 8:2). Forty years! God did not have Israel travel the shortest route to the Promised Land. God seemed in no hurry to give them the land if they weren't ready to live in that land according to his ways.

So, just as he did with the children of Israel, God takes his people on a long wilderness path for a specific reason: "Know then in your heart that as a man disciplines his son, so the LORD your

God disciplines you" (Deut 8:5). God wanted the people of Israel—
and he wants you and me—to recognize that the hard training he
takes us through is one of the best evidences of his loving commitment to us. That's a truth I often miss. Too often I fail to recognize the Lord's training in the hardships I face. Instead, I often
assume that the hard places are a product of my failures or are an
attack of the enemy. But God is bigger than both my failures and
the enemy's efforts. I'm not in the hard places because God is
helpless in the face of their cause. I am in the hard places for my
good and his glory. Yes, God allows us to travel dry places so that
he can refine us.

The Blessings of Dryness

I remember one summer when the lake near a Christian camp our
church often used was drained. What had been a pristine mountain
lake was now an empty hole. A lot of churches—including ours—
cancelled their trips that year. But draining the lake enabled the
camp to make very necessary repairs to the dam and clear out years
of junk from the lake bottom. Is it possible that the dryness that
God allows in my life somehow drains the hydration level so I can
see more clearly what needs to be repaired, make those repairs and
clean out the junk that has settled to the bottom? As a lake drains,
the shallows and the perimeter are exposed first. Then, as the
draining continues, deeper and more central places are exposed.
Will I choose, in seasons of dryness, to trust that God is seeking to
make me holy rather than letting me be satisfied with just looking
holy? That is definitely not my default mode.

I think about the kinds of prayers I've prayed in the dry places.
I am not usually grateful for God's refining work. Far more often I
let him know that I want the water level back where I was comfortable. Yes, I can be so shortsighted. I know what feels good to
me, and I forget what is truly and deeply good. The discomfort and

dissatisfaction of long-term dryness offer a great opportunity for God's Spirit to do a deep, purifying work within us. Dry times expose the vulnerable places in me—the gluttony, lust, greed, envy. You could make your own list. Dry times test my ability to persevere and endure, giving me an opportunity to gain some spiritual muscle. That's all well and good, but the fact remains that hanging in there through the wilderness isn't easy.

Maybe you're like me: I find that my motivation level is often tied to how I am feeling, and dryness feels demotivating. Maybe dryness exposes how selfish even my "spiritual" motives can be. Maybe dryness awakens me to my many disordered thirsts. The same dusty, dry path I've been walking day after day is a hard place to continue to do the work God has entrusted to me. Perhaps, like a tree that has to sink its roots deeper during a drought, I will learn—I will *choose* to learn—to sink my roots down more deeply to where I might find refreshment in God.

PRUNING

One last biblical image that has helped me discern God's direction in the hard places has been that of a branch that has been pruned. Just as seasons of waiting and dryness can prompt prayer, so can those seasons of pruning. John 15—a core passage for me for half my life now—has often spoken to my needs during difficult times. I remember an occasion when verse 2 grabbed my attention: "Every branch that does bear fruit he prunes so that it will be even more fruitful." The question that came to mind was, *So which branches get pruned?* Jesus taught that he prunes the branches that bear fruit. He wasn't talking about pruning fruitless branches.

And what is the aim of the great Gardener when he prunes the branches of your life and mine? He intends to make our lives even more fruitful. This truth nevertheless implies that seasons will come when a branch looks naked—often just after it had been at least a little fruitful. Any pruning experience, whenever it occurs, can leave us feeling a little puny, naked and maybe even robbed. We may also wonder if we'll ever be fruitful again.

I remember a house we once rented. The previous residents had done nothing with the rosebushes in the front yard for years. They were taller than I am—and I'm pretty tall. Our predecessors' theory of rose cultivation was "bigger is better." At the time, I was naive enough to think that we'd have an amazing display of roses in the coming spring. When spring came, however, I don't think any one of those bushes had ten roses the whole season. I realized that those poor rosebushes were so busy trying to keep all their many branches alive that they didn't have anything left for producing roses. So the next winter, I took my three-year-old son out to the front yard with a pair of pruning shears. As I began to prune the rosebushes, I could see the deep worry in his eyes. He was watching Dad kill the rosebushes! When we were done, we had a Dumpster full of rose branches and a few sticks coming out of the dirt here and there. No leaves. And definitely no roses. My son thought our rose story was over. He could not have imagined at the time what would happen come spring: the pruning resulted in incredible beauty. The quality and quantity of the roses we enjoyed were beyond description.

Even today that memory reinforces an important truth about spiritual growth. I want my spiritual life to follow a rhythm like this: I go to God, I grow, I become more and more fruitful, and I keep feeling fruitful every day of my life until the end. I don't factor in or even want to think much about the seasons of necessary pruning, even though only with the Gardener's shears will my life be as fruitful as I want it to be. In other words, the irony is that with the pruning will come answers to my prayers for spiritual fruitfulness. I've asked God to help me grow and be fruitful for his kingdom. I've asked God to enable me to abide deeply in Christ and grow to maturity in him. But in the moment I rarely recognize God's answers to these prayers of mine. Why? Because how I imagine my prayers being answered looks so different from God's wise responses. I'm tempted to believe, for example, that a life of abiding in Christ will always feel consoling, that God will always feel close and that I will always feel certain about my faith. I have learned, though, that pruning experiences cause me to feel less fruitful—if not fruitless—for a season. Even in those times, I can remind myself that greater fruit will result because of this pruning, but I often fail to maintain that perspective. So I'm grateful that God knows what my true desires are when I get stuck in what I feel in the moment.

God's work of pruning is always for our good and for his glory. Pruning, for instance, enables us to move from producing early and lesser-quality fruit to more mature fruit borne from deeper surrender and dependence. Pruning isn't easy. Think of Jesus in the Garden of Gethsemane: he wrestled and struggled in prayer. There was nothing theoretical or cerebral about his questions to God. Instead, Jesus cried out and clawed the ground until he sweat drops of blood. He was not merely modeling certain behaviors for his disciples; Jesus wrestled with all of his strength to surrender to his Father's will. At times we will also struggle, for God often uses seasons of pruning to bring about our cooperation with his plan in our life. And that truth—that journey—is what Jesus modeled for us.

WHAT PRUNING LOOKS LIKE

What do I mean by pruning? One kind of pruning is the experience of outward loss—the loss of relationships, possessions, opportunities, positions of ministry, a sense of respect from others, a sense of status, and the list continues. Such outward losses don't feel like a continuation of our growth. From our in-the-moment vantage point, in fact, pruning feels utterly removed from spiritual growth or fruitfulness of any kind. I'm tempted to follow the farmer who resists pruning an orchard for fear that he will have less produce. A smaller crop for a season will result in a smaller profit, and some farmers can't see beyond that. We believers have the same problem in our Christian life: we assume that growth will always be about just a little more knowledge, a little more influence, a little more recognition. We fail to find a place in our theology of growth for such painful pruning and difficulty surrendering to God's will.

In addition to outward loss, pruning may also involve inward loss—the loss of dreams, plans, hopes or expectations. We might also lose a sense of God's presence. We may lose confidence or clarity about our relationship with the Lord. Yet places like these can deepen our abiding communion with Christ in a way that will one day make our lives more fruitful than we ever dreamed.

Everyone suffers losses, and the pain that accompanies loss prompts many questions, among them, "What does it look like to abide in Christ in those hard places? What does it look like to remain rooted when life doesn't feel good? What does it look like to continue drawing near when God feels far away?"

These questions matter not only to our lives but also to the ministries we participate in and perhaps lead. Are we helping people think well about their own abiding in Christ when they feel disappointed with God? Are we giving easy, simplistic and therefore insensitive answers to people's impossible questions? Are we tempted to tell our struggling friends to just do this or that and things will be better? Are we in a hurry for them to get past this hard season so *we* will feel better? Telling a pruned tree to "just do a little more" is cruel counsel, but we *can* tell the pruned tree, "Abide. Abide deeply. Be restored. Stay rooted. Let God do in you all that God wants to do." The challenge for leaders is that we don't always see a short-term payoff to such counsel in terms of church productivity and church growth the way we tend to measure it.

I knew these truths intellectually, but I was shaken through our hard times. First, as I've described, came the crisis-a-year season of our lives that involved obvious, outward, visible losses, and people around us were easily able to empathize with us in our suffering. At times we were even admired publicly for our heroic faith in God in the midst of the challenges we were facing. To be honest, I kind of enjoyed feeling like a hero of faith and having others admire us. But as we moved into the later nineties, the pruning went from outward and obvious to more inward and invisible—at least to others.

I faced seasons of deep depression, diminished energy and a fading vision for ministry. I experienced deep doubts about how I had understood God up until that point. I wondered if the confident vision of God's nature and his ways that I had held on to and had shared with others was as pure and perfect as I had thought it was: *Maybe I had been misguided, or my mentors in the faith had been mistaken.* Furthermore, such inner pruning didn't elicit as much public empathy as our outward pruning had. I looked—and felt—a lot less like a hero of the faith. I didn't get as much attention or as many kudos from others in these times of inward testing, and that was another part—a big part—of the loss I felt.

Maybe you know something about what I was experiencing: Have you ever looked at your faith walk and wondered, *Is this all?* Can you think of times when your own faith or the faith of your friends seems to have grown drier and crustier over time instead of richer? Does it ever feel as if your faith has become a box you live in that seems to be shrinking over time and confining you, sentencing you to be alone with your pain?

At times God seems to have pruned back my faith structures so that I could grow in my ability to simply trust Jesus. In those places, I wasn't losing faith. I realized later that instead I was losing something of my self-confident understanding of and approach to faith. Perhaps, for instance, I lost confidence in a particular way I quantified, outlined or described faith. From inward hardships like those I've described, I relearn that Jesus is always bigger than my experience of him and always greater than any faith tradition presents him. Always. He is not limited by any human tradition, human expression or human experience. But this truth can make me feel pretty insecure. Somehow I feel safe in my small understanding of Jesus, and I feel threatened by the sense that he is far greater than I'll ever comprehend. Paul prayed that we might be empowered to know the love of Christ that surpasses comprehension (see Eph 3:18-19). But am I willing to allow the Father to enable me to live in relationship with him who is far greater than I can ever fully wrap my mind around? This kind of spacious, unhurried knowledge of God has been one of the resurrection fruits following the death of certain understandings of God.

A SIMPLE INVITATION

Returning to John 15, I was struck there by the idea that a branch that has been pruned has a single primary need—to remain well connected to the vine. When we experience loss that seems to diminish who we are, we need more than ever to remain deeply connected to God through Christ. Unlike trees that have no choice, we who are God's children have the ability to choose between responding to God or resisting him, between saying yes to him and saying no. Will we keep abiding in the One who has allowed us to experience loss, who uses our times of loss as pruning places in our lives?

We may be tempted to question God's goodness in such hard seasons, but F. B. Meyer, an itinerant evangelist and minister in the late nineteenth and early twentieth centuries, helps us here:

> *God always keeps the discipline of sorrow in His own hands.* Our Lord said, "My Father is the husbandman." His hand holds the pruning knife. His eye watches the crucible. His gentle touch is on the pulse while the operation is in progress. . . . The moments are carefully allotted. The severity of the test is exactly determined by the reserves of grace and strength that are lying unrecognized within, but will be sought for and used beneath the severe pressure of pain.[4]

Meyer understood. Whenever we find ourselves in a season of waiting or dryness or pruning, and therefore feeling weak and weary, we can learn to be patient as God sensitizes us to the reality of his ever-present grace in the darkness. When we keep our focus on God like that, we can grow in grace despite—even because of—the hardship.

UNHURRIED TIME

1. Describe the most recent time you found yourself in a spiritual waiting room. How did you feel about God? How did you feel about yourself? What do you think might have been God's invitation to you in this perhaps unwelcome place of unhurry?

2. At what point has your life with God gone from feeling refreshing and close to feeling dry and distant? In what ways, if any, did this change seem to be about misguided choices or missteps on your part? In what ways might God have been inviting you to sink your roots deeper into him by drying up a familiar, comfortable place where you may have, in fact, become stuck?

3. Think about some of the losses you have experienced in your life. Describe them in terms of pruning that produced more or better fruit later on.

4. In what ways is God inviting you to draw near to him in the midst of whatever hardships you are now facing? What honest prayer do you want to share with the One who loves you more than you can imagine?

MATURITY

Growing Up Takes Time

As I've been writing this book, I passed the one-third-century mark as a Christian: I have followed Jesus for thirty-three-and-a-third years since I encountered him in my high school years. Of course I've followed more closely in some seasons than in others. One of the questions I've asked myself is, *Have I been growing for thirty-three years with Jesus, or have I sometimes lived the same year over and over again, covering the same ground year after year?* I'm saddened to think about those seasons when I made little progress depending more on Jesus or—even by the Spirit's power—surrendering more to Jesus or following him more wholeheartedly.

It's hard to argue with the idea that growth happens over time. You might be able to grow a turnip to maturity in a couple of months, but that's not true for people. It may take nine months for a baby to fully develop in her mother's womb, but it takes years for that baby to reach physical maturity, and longer still to reach emotional, relational and spiritual maturity. And when it comes to our spiritual life, many of us are tempted to look for shortcuts to growth and maturity. Some of us, for instance, assume that the main cause of spiritual maturity comes through either doing more ministry for God or gathering, organizing and remembering more and more biblical, theological and spiritual knowledge. In *Practice Resurrection*, author Eugene Peterson points out that "maturity cannot be hurried, programmed, or tinkered with. There are no steroids available for growing up in Christ more quickly. Impatient shortcuts land us in the dead ends of immaturity."[1] In fact, the impatience with which we seek to achieve spiritual maturity is implicit evidence of our immaturity. Brother Lawrence observed about a particularly enthusiastic sister that "it seems like her heart is in the right place, but she wants to advance faster than grace would allow. You don't become a saint in a day!"[2] Are you, like that dear sister and me, trying sometimes to progress faster than the pace of grace?

Baron Friedrich von Hügel, spiritual director to Evelyn Underhill and many others, shared what an early spiritual director in his life said about growth in character:

> When, at eighteen, I made up my mind to go into moral and religious training, the great soul and mind who took me in hand—a noble Dominican—warned me: "You want to grow in virtue, to serve God, to love Christ? Well, you will grow in and attain to these things if you will make them a slow and sure, an utterly real, a mountain step-plod and ascent, willing to have to camp for weeks or months in spiritual desolation, darkness and emptiness at different stages in your march and growth. All demand for constant light, for ever the best—the best to your own feeling, all attempt at eliminating or minimizing the cross and trial, is so much soft folly and puerile trifling."[3]

Along with stretching my comprehension to its limits, von Hügel reminds me that growth in goodness is not fast. It is not a sprint followed by additional sprints. Growth in goodness—in Christlikeness—is a steady, day-by-day, footstep-after-footstep journey. To our overstimulated hearts and minds, that path may sound boring. Perhaps we assume that our relationship with God is supposed to be a continuous honeymoon where we always feel God and always feel good. Any of us who have been married even a few years know that is an unrealistic expectation. Yet we also recognize the potential places of growth and maturity that can be richer and deeper than the surface excitement of the early moments of marriage.

Not only is growth in goodness slower than we wish, but it is also difficult to define. I remember having a conversation about spiritual maturity with fellow church staff members, many of whom were older than me. We were trying to figure out together how spiritual maturity worked and, even more, how to describe or define it. Our conclusion? None of us had a crisp definition. We agreed that spiritual depth measured in terms of merely knowing things isn't enough, but we didn't know how to offer a more full-bodied description. Many years later, I'm hardly ready to write the definitive word on spiritual growth and maturity, but I would like to share some of what I've been learning.

A simple idea about changes in organizational settings in Paul Hersey and Ken Blanchard's *Management of Organizational Behavior* has helped me in my reflections on the theme of spiritual maturity and how it develops. They suggest that

> changes in knowledge are the easiest to make, followed by changes in attitudes. Attitude structures differ from knowledge structures in that *they are emotionally charged in a positive or negative way.* Changes in behavior are significantly more difficult and time consuming than either of the two previous levels. But the implementation of group or organizational performance change is perhaps the most difficult and time consuming.[4]

It strikes me that we could think about spiritual growth and maturity in each one of these categories: knowledge, attitude, personal behavior and communal behavior. Since I have lived my adult life in the evangelical Protestant tradition, for instance, I experienced a focus on growing our knowledge and improving our behavior. I don't remember much practical attention given to our attitude. Over time, though, I have been impressed that Jesus focused much of his attention on matters of attitude, matters of heart. One of the barriers that hinders our growth is that we learn something and then just try to make it happen in our lives without much reflection on the resistance such ideas can stir within us. Within me are hidden, if not ignored, resistances to the good practice, behavior or habit that I'm trying to establish, and that is one reason why behavioral changes don't stick. In fact, certain assumptions, beliefs, expectations and desires exist that are energized not by the Spirit of God but by inner distortions of desire shaped by the God-disregarding world in which I've grown up. I fail to make progress when such places of the heart and mind are left untouched in my efforts to change my behaviors.

I think of the teachings of Jesus, especially some of his parables. In the parable of the sower, for example, Jesus described the outcome of seed planted in four different places—hard ground, shallow terrain, a weed-infested field and fertile soil. What he was focusing on is the heart and attitude of people who hear the gospel.

After mentioning the "hard ground" where the seed has no chance to grow at all, Jesus mentions the seed planted "on the rocky ground" or in shallow soil as representing "the ones who receive the word with joy when they hear it, but they have no root. They believe for a while, but in the time of testing they fall away" (Lk 8:13). Initial enthusiasm and delight result in rapid growth, but the challenges and hardships that come their way cause them to quickly question what they hear. There is little perseverance in their perspective. Perhaps they were expecting nothing but joy and are therefore surprised by experiences of adversity. The shallowness of the soil corresponds to the superficiality of their heart's response to the truth of the gospel they hear.

Other seed falls not on rocky ground but among thorns, and those thorns represent "those who hear, but as they go on their way they are choked by life's worries, riches and pleasures, and they do not mature" (Lk 8:14). These seeds don't mature because the young plants are overwhelmed by such weeds as anxiety, greed and lust. These heart realities prevent the full growth and fruitfulness of God's Word and God's ways in people's lives. They make the mistake of thinking that their life comes from what they acquire and possess or consume and use. Such a perspective is unseasoned and immature.

But then there is seed that finds its way into fertile soil. The seed grew, "came up and yielded a crop, a hundred times more than was sown. . . . The seed on good soil stands for those with a noble and good heart, who hear the word, retain it, and by persevering produce a crop" (Lk 8:8, 15). Again, notice the noble and good heart—the soil—that resulted in the fruitfulness and maturing of this seed. Maturity takes time; it requires unhurried perseverance. Fruitfulness comes in no other way. The only effective response to God's Word is noble-hearted, pure and weed-resistant. This fertile soil is a heart able to hold on tight against discouragement: it perseveres and never gives up.

How Leaders Help Us Mature

It is crucial to note that none of us followers of Christ matures on our own. In fact, God uses all kinds of people to help us along the way. What can these fellow believers do to encourage and support us along the way? And what might we do to foster growth in the lives of those God has brought into our life?

For starters, Paul reminds us of this important truth:

Christ himself gave the apostles, the prophets, the evange-
lists, the pastors and teachers, to equip his people for works
of service, so that the body of Christ may be built up until we
all reach unity in the faith and in the knowledge of the Son of
God and become mature, attaining to the whole measure of
the fullness of Christ. (Eph 4:11-13)

These leaders are a gift of Christ to his people, a gift that enables
each one of us to better offer our gift for the good of the body. I am
grateful for such gifts, for the men and women God has used to
help clear obstacles in my path, to show me the way, to help me
find healing, and to encourage and enable me to contribute to the
good of his people. Certain God-appointed individuals have helped
me journey to places of a deeper faith in God and richer intimacy
with Christ. These people have, in fact, helped me grow more into
the fullness of Christ. What great gifts God gives.

One believer who has helped many others grow is Shirley Carter
Hughson, who served for many years as an Anglican abbot in New
York. Listen to what he said about the unhurried work of helping
others become more fruitful:

I am sure that when St. Paul spoke of "the fruit of the Spirit,"
he had in mind such processes as we find in nature. A tree
which brings forth good fruit is able to do so because over
many years it has been brought under the influence of cultivation, fertilization, sunshine, rain, caressing winds, spraying
and cleansing from blight, and so it acquires the power to
bear good fruit. A farmer cannot get this result by suddenly
becoming very busy for a season and doing these things.

Wise leaders understand this principle: they realize the necessity of consistent, ongoing, and patient teaching; they un-

derstand that teaching people how to draw on the grace of God is not a task to accomplish but a relationship they tend. With Christian leadership based on that principle, individuals grow in their ability to resist the power of false ways of living and learn how to "follow the steady leading of the Holy Spirit."[5]

I am also hopeful that such leaders will stop using people to further their own ministry goals and instead, by serving these people, enable them to offer their own God-given ministries for the good of the kingdom. God longs that each one of us would come to share in the life of the Son, growing up into the fullness of who Jesus is. Leaders aren't so much directly responsible for maturing in the body, but for preparing all of God's people to take responsibility for our own mutual maturing. That is an inspiring and—without God's help—overwhelming goal.

And perhaps one of the most challenging elements of this work is praying for those we lead. In his writing to the Colossians, Paul mentions Epaphras, a colleague who was "always wrestling in prayer for you, that you may stand firm in all the will of God, mature and fully assured" (4:12). Many of us in leadership roles and positions overemphasize the power of our public work of teaching, planning, preaching, organizing, counseling and so on, and we underemphasize the power of our quiet work of simply praying. I'm not so much talking about circumstantial prayers where we ask God to somehow change something in our situation or in others', but about soul prayers where we focus our attention on what's happening in a person's heart, on what's happening in his or her relationship with Jesus and with others. Our work of making disciples gains traction as, like Epaphras, we steadily wrestle in prayer for fellow believers so that they are able to stand solid where they have been tentative and unsteady (Col 4:12).

Eugene Peterson, a gift of God to many Christian leaders, makes a similar point. He has said much about the need for Christian leaders who will keep focusing their attention on helping the people of God mature. Peterson told of a pastor who had been moving from church to church, perhaps looking for new challenges to work on and solve in short order. When he pointed out to that pastor "that the persevering, patient, unhurried work of growing up in Christ has occupied the center of the church's life for centuries," Peterson says, this pastor "dismissed me. He needed, he said, a challenge. I took it from his tone and manner that a challenge was by definition something that could be met and accomplished in forty days. That's all the time, after all, that it took Jesus."[6] All I can say is that, when I look back over my few decades of ministry, I am not most excited about any short-term gain or in-the-moment success of some program. Instead I celebrate the lives of men and women with whom I've been honored to share the life of Christ and who have grown their roots deep into Jesus. It has taken time—a long time—but it has been time well spent.

I recently had the opportunity to visit Northern California wine country. During the trip, we spoke with the owner of a vineyard and winery. Brice was kind enough to give us a private audience since his winery did not have a public tasting room. Five years earlier, he had learned about "dry farming" from some fellow wine makers in France. Dry farming involves no artificial irrigation, but relies only on water that comes naturally in that particular setting. (We might say, "Only the water that God provides.")

He shared that they made a plan spanning a few years to wean the plants off of their dependency on the drip irrigation system. He talked about the vines being "addicted" to artificial watering. He mentioned that vines that grow with irrigation develop a relatively small, onion-shaped root ball since they don't need to reach any farther for the water they need. His belief is that a healthy vine has as much mass in its root system as it does in the plant that is above ground, but this does not happen with drip-irrigated vines.

He was willing to try this experiment even though very few others had done so in the region. The cost of this transition was significant. In the first year that they reduced the artificial water supply, their yield dropped by 45 percent. It took a few years for their yield to come back close to what they were getting from their irrigated vineyard. He shared that now that the transition is complete, they still have a slightly lower yield than before but they are getting a much higher quality of fruit. And one benefit of this transition came in a year when a heavy rain came early in the growing season and caused most vineyards to lose their entire crop to rot. The fruit of his vines, though, consistently matured sooner in the season so that they were able to harvest their crop before this rain hit.

My mind spun as I thought about the implications of this story in relation to the experience of many Christians I know. Many are quite dependent on someone else (a pastor, a mentor, a teacher) providing them with nourishment from outside. As a result, their root system is relatively underdeveloped. They have not learned, nor often been expected, to stretch out their roots to seek re-freshment and nourishment for themselves. If churches and ministries were to redesign their efforts to be more intentional about helping Christians find their nourishment in Jesus for themselves, there might be complaints and a loss of "fruit" for a season (or a few seasons). But what might happen to the quality of these men's and women's lives as a result? How might they come to be so well rooted that they would no longer be dependent on someone else for their growth and could, in fact, become a source of nourishment and refreshment for others? Such a "dry farming" experiment in a local church or ministry would be a worthy one.[7]

Such an experiment might look like Quaker author Thomas

Kelly's description of believers being enabled to enter into "the
simplicity of the trusting child, the simplicity of the children of
God." He continued:

> It is the simplicity that lies beyond complexity. It is the na-
> ïveté that is the yonder side of sophistication. It is the be-
> ginning of spiritual maturity, which comes after the awkward
> age of religious busyness for the Kingdom of God—yet how
> many are caught, and arrested in development, within this
> adolescent development of the soul's growth![8]

I pray for leaders who will help us move through the hyperactivity of spiritual adolescence into fruitfully unhurried work.

UNDERSTANDING SPIRITUAL MATURITY

Jesus issued a very straightforward invitation to maturity in his
Sermon on the Mount: "Be perfect, therefore, as your heavenly
Father is perfect" (Mt 5:48). Though I'm tempted to hear these
words with ears of perfectionism, I can instead choose to hear them
as an invitation into transforming communion with the Holy One
who is my Father in heaven. Maturity here isn't a performance I try
to perfect apart from God but for him. Instead, spiritual maturity is
the welcome fruit that comes as a result of living and lingering
with the Father who loves me. Consequently, maturity is not measured by my own—or by any other—*human* standard, but by the
loving perfection of our heavenly Father. So of course such spiritual maturity doesn't come in an instant.

The writer of Hebrews issued these words of warning:

> Though by this time you ought to be teachers, you need
> someone to teach you the elementary truths of God's word all
> over again. You need milk, not solid food! Anyone who lives
> on milk, being still an infant, is not acquainted with the

teaching about righteousness. But solid food is for the mature, who by constant use have trained themselves to distinguish good from evil. (Heb 5:12-14)

In my evangelical experience, teachers have defined *milk* and *meat* as, respectively, easier, basic teachings and harder, more advanced teachings. These definitions seem to only address understanding, whereas both milk and meat here are related to "teaching about righteousness." The spiritually mature are those who are able to take in solid food, digest it and, as a result, grow in righteousness. With consistent practice, they have also become more able to discern what is truly good and what is actually evil. They are no longer infants who put just anything into their mouths, but adults who can—and should—know what is healthy and good.

Then, calling believers to move along toward spiritual maturity, the writer of Hebrews issues the charge to "not [lay] again the foundation of repentance from acts that lead to death, and of faith in God" (Heb 6:1). The author addresses other foundational lessons for spiritual maturity, but I want to briefly highlight two. First, in the early stages of following Jesus, we need to orient ourselves away from death and toward life. This basic and necessary shift happens when we are taught not only *what* to obey but also *how* to obey. The other basic foundation stone is, simply, trusting God. We mature as we grow in our ability to trust our trustworthy Father. This trust permeates a mature believer's assumptions, expectations and deep beliefs.

Like the author of Hebrews, Paul talks about wisdom for those who are *mature,* wisdom that is "not the wisdom of this age or of the rulers of this age, who are coming to nothing. No, we declare God's wisdom, a mystery that has been hidden and that God destined for our glory before time began" (1 Cor 2:6-7). A person with mature understanding has been freed over time from bondage to the conventional wisdom of the culture or the so-called experts of our time; a spiritually mature understanding appreciates God's wisdom that has been hidden but is revealed more and more to eyes that are ready to see. A spiritually mature believer is also able to discern the difference between the "quick guarantee" promises of the popular authorities and the deeper, unhurried wisdom of a God who hides true wisdom "from sophisticates and know-it-alls, but [spells] them out clearly to ordinary people" (Mt 11:25-26 *The Message*). God has commanded through Paul that we "stop thinking like children. In regard to evil be infants, but in your thinking be *adults*" (1 Cor 14:20, emphasis mine). Maturity involves growing beyond the naiveté of childhood but retaining a childlike innocence in relation to evil.

ATTITUDES AND PERSPECTIVES

So what perspective or attitude do I see in the life of a spiritually growing follower of Christ? The writings of the apostle John speak to that matter.

In his first letter, John said, "I am writing to you, fathers, because you know him who is from the beginning. I am writing to you, young men, because you have overcome the evil one. I write to you, dear children, because you know the Father" (1 Jn 2:13-14). Fathers have come to know their eternal Father and are a little further along in the journey of faith. Christian maturity comes with an intimate and deep knowledge of a loving Father. These mature believers are able to encourage and care for those just starting their journey, enabling them to grow confident about the Father's love and care. These fathers in the faith can also counsel newer believers struggling with false ways of life, encouraging them to dwell more and more in the freedom and vitality of God's presence.

In his letter to the Philippians, Paul wrote: "I press on toward the goal to win the prize for which God has called me heavenward in Christ Jesus. All of us, then, who are mature should take such a view of things. And if on some point you think differently, that too God will make clear to you" (3:14-15). In other words, a mature perspective on life can be measured by an increasingly single and sharp focus on Jesus Christ himself. Earlier, Paul shared his own attitude about the many good things in his life:

> Whatever were gains to me I now consider loss for the sake of Christ. What is more, I consider everything a loss because of the surpassing worth of knowing Christ Jesus my Lord, for whose sake I have lost all things. I consider them garbage, that I may gain Christ. (Phil 3:7-8)

Maturity is the fruit of a long and focused journey toward realizing that everything good can only be truly enjoyed in the only One who is truly good. The ability to more fully abide in Jesus and appreciate every good blessing is unhurried fruit of a believer's journey toward wholeness.

Again, in line with Paul's teaching, the writer of Hebrews urges believers to journey through life with "our eyes [fixed] on Jesus, the pioneer and perfecter of faith. For the joy set before him he endured the cross, scorning its shame, and sat down at the right hand of the throne of God" (Heb 12:2). Jesus is the One who got us started on the journey of faith, and he is the One who will bring us to full maturity. Mature faith focuses its gaze more and more on Jesus himself, allowing him to fill the horizon of one's perspectives, expectations and assumptions.

A LIFE THAT LEADS TO MATURITY

Having reflected on the understanding and attitude of a maturing Christian, consider now what their behavior looks like. We'll start with a conversation Jesus had.

When a wealthy young man asked Jesus just what good thing he needed to do to guarantee he would have eternal life, Jesus said, "If you want to be *perfect*, go, sell your possessions and give to the poor, and you will have treasure in heaven. Then come, follow me" (Mt 19:21, emphasis mine). Moving toward maturity in our spiritual journey may invite us into the willing loss of good things to which we have become attached. If we have an inordinate attachment to our wealth or our possessions, God just might invite us to release them so that our hands are open and able to receive him. We approach spiritual maturity as we walk along a path of such loving surrender to the Lord.

Providing additional wise words for our journey on that path, James highlights the strategic importance of watching what we say: "We all stumble in many ways. Anyone who is never at fault in what they say is perfect, able to keep their whole body in check" (Jas 3:2). Maturing in our faith is demonstrated when we speak to others in a way that is full of grace and under the Spirit's control. When we are mature in our faith, our words express love instead of control, kindness instead of harshness, and exuberant joy instead of despair or hopelessness.

Furthermore, in his first letter, John reminds us that "there is no fear in love. But perfect love drives out fear, because fear has to do with punishment. The one who fears is not made perfect in love" (1 Jn 4:18). Those who are "made perfect in love" are mature believers. These followers of Christ also experience a growing sense of being loved, and this realization is evident in their being more loving with other people. Yet too often evangelical believers tend to measure spiritual maturity in terms of things we know over who and how we love. Perhaps fear is at the heart of this misguided use of an inaccurate gauge. As our hearts are more at home in the One who loves us most, we come to live more wholly and more holy.

Spiritual Formation in a Church

Having thought about how Christian leaders may or may not help the rest of us grow in our relationship with Jesus, let's consider what spiritual formation tends to look like in various churches and ministries. Most church leaders these days, if asked what their strategy is for helping their people grow up in Christ, will talk about their spiritual formation plan, strategy or program. What do these tend to look like?

A change of title. Sometimes a church takes an existing position (pastor/director of Christian education or small groups or adults) or program (adult Sunday school or discipleship) and simply changes the label to include the phrase *spiritual formation*. The leader gets a new title, a new business card and a new plate on the office door. The group or program gets a new name. The assumption may be that a change of name will result in a change in substance, but the transformation rarely happens—and that fact shouldn't surprise anyone. Relabeling may make people try an old something with the thought that it's now new, but eventually everyone realizes nothing has really changed.

A change of curriculum. A ministry may introduce a spiritual-formation-themed sermon series or start using spiritual formation curriculum in their small groups, youth group or adult classes. Pastors may recommend books on spiritual formation themes or even provide them in a church bookstore or library. While this approach is an improvement over the name-change option, the fact is that learning information *about* spiritual formation may or may not bring *actual* transformation. Increasing knowledge is important in spiritual formation, but it is not the whole of it. In fact, our tendency to focus so much on the delivery of content in our Christian gatherings may be having the unintended effect of training people to become increasingly comfortable with undigested and unpracticed insights. Think about highly involved Christians who hear a sermon on the weekend, perhaps attend a small group with a curriculum about spiritual formation and maybe even read a book on their own time. This may lead to the unanalyzed and perhaps unspoken idea that putting into practice all that they have learned is impossible. Many good insights can overwhelm us and become ideas we merely agree with rather than guidelines for a Spirit-guided and Spirit-empowered way of life. Practiced experience in the way of Christ takes time.

Adding another specialization. The approach of adding another specialization involves establishing a ministry that actually provides—for those people who are especially drawn to it—some level of training, experiences and mentoring in spiritual formation. Such a church regards spiritual formation as one more way to get people involved in the church according to their personal interests. So spiritual formation is one more offering on a church's ever-lengthening buffet table, and it competes against other specialties like Bible study, missions, evangelism, intercession and small groups for the time and attention of church attendees. People pick what they like and stay away from what they don't. This approach tends to be rooted in a (perhaps unconscious) consumerist vision of church. It may also assume that those people who will be interested in spiritual formation will be introverts, more reflective and quiet than, say, the person who chooses evangelism. Sadly, in this model, spiritual formation is not regarded as a universal invitation or a growth process for every believer or the soil in which *everything* in the church grows.

Personally holy, vocationally unholy. The phrase "personally holy, vocationally unholy" comes from Eugene Peterson's *Under the Unpredictable Plant,* where he talks about leaders who experience *personal* spiritual transformation through intimacy with Christ but it seems to have little impact on either the actual work of ministry or how it is approached. There may, of course, be a change in curriculum—a change in what the leader preaches and teaches—but there is little difference in any of the methods of ministry. Personal spiritual refreshment, renewal and transformation do not appear to result in a different way of leading. One set of values guides the life, while another set appears to guide the ministry.

The spiritual transformation of ministry structures. Here, the transformation that begins in the life of the leader begins to change the actual *how* of ministry. Transformation is not limited to a change in teaching or preaching content, in curriculum for small groups or age-level ministries, or in specialized offerings to interested participants. Transformation extends to places of strategic and programmatic planning, policy and financial decision making, as well as to how leaders and leadership teams function together. The power structures of the church operate less independently and with greater dependence on God. Leaders make space and allow generous time for spiritual practices in their planning and decision-making meetings. Questions I've found helpful here include, "In your life and ministry, how do prayer and planning relate? Are they intimate allies, casual acquaintances or relative strangers? Do you turn to prayer as your last resort or as your first impulse?"

A church board, for instance, may have been accustomed to opening with a few moments of prayer or devotion, an activity that, at the unspoken level, most in the room realize isn't the *important* part of the meeting, but a *prelude* to the important part—to the decisions to be made, events to be planned and so on. The feeling seems to be that it's good to pray a little before moving on to the planning and decision making. When this church becomes interested in genuine spiritual transformation, such meetings will look very different. That board begins to spend significant time together reflecting on Scripture and letting God use it as a source of actual guidance for decisions and plans. The board also gives time to listen to God in prayer as they bring particular people and specific concerns before him. These members of the board expect that such attention to God will make them wiser, more buoyant in attitude, more united in spiritual vision, more creative in response to practical challenges and more encouraged about implementing what is planned. This board experiences a sense of deeply felt need for God's intervention in their shared work if their ministry together is to reflect his intentions and desires.

Conclusion

I hear a lot of talk about "deep" when it comes to growing in Christ. My sense of what the average evangelical Christian means by *deep* is theologically, biblically, doctrinally rich and profound, and this is probably measured mostly in terms of cognitive content. But there are other ways to measure depth. There is soul depth, referring to the dynamics in my life with God and with other people. There is spiritual depth, meaning the level of my personal receptivity to and engagement with God in the moment-to-moment living of life. There is heart depth: I am more emotionally responsive to God and others as well as more willing to show my love for God by obeying him. Are we open to God's bringing such depth to every facet of our lives? Will we enter into deep soul work, deep interaction with God, deep sharing of our lives together and deep engagement with the non-followers in our lives? Will we seek *life* deep and not settle for just *intellect* deep?

An unhurried vision of growth and maturity brings freedom and encouragement because we have a whole lifetime to grow. I don't have to keep living the same year of my Christian life over and over again with little actual personal transformation. I am invited into a renewing and deepening awareness of God's love as well as new ways of expressing that love in my ministry to others. I don't have to be the same person spiritually in five years that I am today. My roots can slowly and surely sink deeper into all that God has for me. New branches will grow, branches that were never there before, because old branches have been pruned away. I can trust that God intends my life to be more fruitful than I can imagine. I can grow more confident that "Christian maturity is not a matter of doing more for God; it is God doing more in and through us. Immaturity is noisy with anxiety-fueled self-importance. Maturity is quietly content to pursue a life of obedient humility."[9] This is a vision I pray will take root in your heart and encourage you as you steadily make your way along the path God is taking you.

UNHURRIED TIME

1. What does impatience to grow spiritually look like in your life? In the lives of others around you? In what ways does this impatience hinder more than help your progress?

2. When did you first begin to trust in and follow Jesus? What did those early seasons of growth and maturing look like for you? What did seasons of being a bit stuck look like?

3. If someone asked you, "How do I know if I'm maturing as a follower of Jesus?" what would your response be?

Spiritual Practices
for Unhurrying

I remember a day of solitude that happened over twenty years ago like it was yesterday. It was one of those moments that has marked the rest of my life. I was a student at Fuller Seminary, and in one of my classes we were given three hours to be alone and quiet with God at a nearby large church property. I wrote in my journal that day:

> Lord, I don't know what to do with three hours alone with you. I want to know you more, but I don't like the way this time makes me feel so out of control. Please quiet my mind and heart so that I can pay attention to you. Give me courage to respond to you.
>
> As I begin, I sense you reminding me that you are my Father—my *Abba*. I need to let that soak in. I'm not sure what to do with this. After sitting at a picnic table for a while, I have a thought that just will not go away: *Go swing on the swing set*. It is persistent. I feel resistance rise up within me: *I don't want to swing on the swings. I'm a grown man, and that would be humiliating*. Besides, the only swings I saw here were

made for five-year-olds, not twenty-nine-year-olds. I'm not even sure they will hold my weight.

I try to discern the source of this unwelcome thought. Where is it coming from? Is the evil one trying to distract me? What would *he* gain from this? Nothing. Is this my own idea? Hardly! I'd be too embarrassed to do anything like this. Lord, if this is you, what are you doing? This feels ridiculous. I'm afraid of what the mothers of small children over in that playground will think, but I can't think of any other reason not to respond. So I will sit on the swings, even if it is only out of sheer obedience to you.

Well, I did it. I sat on the swings, feeling foolish and uncomfortable. As I sat there and began to swing back and forth, another strong thought of my own came to mind: *I don't like being thought of as a child. I don't like the feeling of being out of control or not in charge. I don't want to be powerless or weak.*

Almost as though the conversation were happening in my heart, I sensed God say, "Those who come to me must come as children and embrace me as *Abba*." Then, instead of responding with humble gratitude for this precious expression of God's love for me, I felt angry. In fact, I found myself praying, "The idea of addressing you as Daddy feels irreverent and flippant. I've assumed that people who talk to you like that are taking you lightly and treating you like a buddy. But now I am beginning to realize that I'm more concerned about myself and my reputation than I am about you and your honor.

"Forgive me, Abba. Daddy, I can see that I am your beloved little one. Being little before you is good news. I am grateful for your tender and protective affection. No one has ever had an earthly father better than you."

Let me share a few spiritual practices that have helped me in my journey toward living a more unhurried life in communion with Jesus. The most important for me have been the classic practices of solitude, silence and prayer.

EXTENDED PERSONAL COMMUNION WITH GOD (EPC)

On the day I ended up swinging and being captured by the deep love of Abba for me, I was practicing what my mentor, Wayne Anderson, called times of *Extended Personal Communion with God*, or EPC for short. I liked that because "solitude and silence" has sometimes sounded rather empty and lonely to my still-learning ears. Wayne's term was warmer and more inviting. He encouraged us, one day each month, to get away for at least a few hours to just *be* in God's presence. It was a habit he had been practicing for many years. Rationale for this rhythm came from Elton Trueblood:

> One rare but powerful item of discipline is the requirement that the recruit of the company undertake a personal experience of solitude at least once a month. This is patterned consciously on the experience of Christ who periodically went alone, even at the price of temporary separation from the needs of His fellows. The justification of aloneness is not that of refined self-indulgence, but rather a consequent enrichment of one's subsequent contribution. A person who is always available is not worth enough when he *is* available. Everyone engaged in public life will realize the extreme difficulty to getting away each month for a period of five or six hours, but the difficulty is not a good reason for rejecting the discipline. It is the men and women who find it hardest to get away who need the redemptive solitude most sorely.[1]

As I mentioned in chapter six, Jesus would sometimes invite his disciples away from the demands of ministry and take them with him to be alone and quiet in retreat. This invitation from Jesus appears in the Gospel of Mark: "Come with me by yourselves to a quiet place and get some rest" (6:31). I can't think of a stronger rationale than this for encouraging people who are busy in any kind of ministry or work to set aside regular times for EPC. We might resist such a rhythm out of fear that it would somehow reduce our productivity. We can, instead, see it as an opportunity to be refreshed and empowered by God for the good work he has given us to do. Then, renewed, revitalized and ready once again, we can return to the good work given to us.

Now, however, convinced of the value of my EPC days, I face a different challenge. I find myself tempted to pack my EPC days with lots of spiritual activities like reading, journaling, ministry preparation, recreation activities and so on. I want to make the most of the time by doing as many good spiritual things as possible. And, yes, when the number of spiritual exercises I get done is my gauge, my retreat days can end up being just as scheduled and hurried as any other day. But the invitation of EPC is, for a time, to be alone and quiet in the welcoming presence of Jesus. That's how he measures it. We offer him uncluttered space and unhurried time during which we choose to simply be present to him, to listen for his voice or seek to be attentive to his presence.

Often when I lead EPC days for groups of Christian leaders, the question surfaces: "How do you actually practice solitude and silence?" I have learned to reframe the question: "What you are basically asking is 'How do you *do* being?'" It sounds silly to say it that way, but we practice solitude by remaining alone and silence by staying quiet. This is not easy, but it is fairly straightforward and a very worthwhile goal. We trust God's Spirit to help us linger in a place that feels like a waste of time to some part of us. But an EPC is to be more like a Sabbath day than a workday. It is a day not measured by productivity (even spiritual productivity), but by rest, creative expression, communion and other restorative ways of investing time.

This practice of EPC is a challenge for many of us. We tend to find disciplines of "doing" easier than disciplines of "not doing" or even "undoing." Yet EPC invites us to cease from our many words and many works so as to make little spaces to notice God in our lives. By ceasing, for a time, from my normal patterns of being in conversation and community with others, I am able to hear his voice and sense (or at least trust) his presence. These open spaces eventually help to calm my inner anxiety and slow down my drivenness. Those impulses that drive me might complain like impatient adolescents as I enter into EPC times, but when I resist them with persistence, these voices eventually give up on their incessant urgings to keep me moving so fast.

The discipline of EPC gives me the opportunity to set aside a time and a place to be attentive, receptive and, by God's grace, responsive to whatever he initiates. Sometimes he chooses to just be with me in the solitary quiet without seeming to say or do anything. And might that not be a sign of intimacy, like a longtime married couple who can sit quietly in the same room without feeling a compulsive need to fill the silence with words?

A good portion of my ministry is the mentoring of Christians (many of them leaders) who want to learn to live an unhurried life. I help them learn to slow down enough to listen to God rather than running past him. I provide day retreats that are, in part, decompression space. Many of the retreats I have attended are quite full of words—good words spoken by good people with good intentions. But I believe that opportunities for unhurried time and uncluttered space with God are often an even greater gift than any words anyone can say. In that kind of silence, our inward driven pace can slow down a bit. We can sense in our heart the peace of God sinking in and the joy of the Lord rising up, and there we find it easier to distinguish God's voice, his direction, and his counsel from all the other voices, directions and counsel that surround us. Such spiritual direction is, in part, a process of recovering from our addiction to hurry and drivenness.

This discussion calls to mind Jesus' teaching on prayer when he urged us to stop "babbling like pagans, for they think they will be heard because of their many words. Do not be like them, for your Father knows what you need before you ask him" (Mt 6:7-8). Jesus was not recommending silence here, but a reduction of words. I've prayed with followers of Jesus from many traditions. When it comes to those of us in the body of Christ who are of the evangelical persuasion, we are, by comparison, among the wordiest and most hurried when we pray. But Jesus once pointed out that it is the pagans who don't know the Father who ramble on and on, assuming that the more words they say, the better their prayer and therefore the more likely God will hear and answer.

I don't believe that about God or about lengthy prayers, so why do I tend to use a lot of words when I pray? Do I forget that my loving Father already knows what I need before I ask? Do I somehow believe that I need to inform the Almighty of something he does not yet know? And in what specific ways would my prayers be simpler if I truly believed that God both knows and cares about what I need? So, when I pray, I might do well to begin with no words at first, but instead to simply remember God's presence with me, by his Spirit and with his great favor. God wants good for me. May I remember that truth and rest in the fact that I don't need to either inform God or convince him about anything. I just need to ask him.

Whenever I talk about my ongoing recovery from my hurried way of life, I realize that this practice of EPC contributes much to my improving spiritual health. When I am alone and quiet in God's loving presence, I find out just how hurried inside I really am. Furthermore, God reminds me that I have—by his grace—made great progress. When I first began this practice, I sometimes felt ready to be done after just thirty minutes or an hour. Since then I've realized that I was trying too hard: I was trying to make solitude and silence happen rather than simply receiving them as a gracious gift from my loving Father. And on occasion I found myself trying to impress God with my heroic commitment to carving out time with him. But wearing such a mask takes a lot of energy. Over time, I have discovered that it helps if I think of an EPC day as simply an opportunity to be together with Jesus, my good Friend (see Jn 15:15).

Sometimes it helps me to practice this discipline of EPC in conjunction with others. On such a day, I'll often build in some blocks of solitude (just Christ and me) and some blocks of community (sharing Christ with another). This accountability and companionship have proven fruitful in my efforts to establish a rhythm in my life that includes resting with the Lord, and he has blessed those individuals who join me. We have even been blessed by being alone with God together, quiet before God in one another's presence.

So what can you do with a few hours alone and quiet in God's presence? Here are a few things that have helped me:

- Start with no agenda—or acknowledge whatever agenda you may have brought to the time. Whenever we go before God, it is helpful to acknowledge the unanswered questions or unclear direction we've brought to our time with him. Perhaps he'll meet us in regard to the specifics that are on our hearts or minds, but maybe he has other issues he wishes to raise with us. We need to listen with an open mind to notice where he may be leading us. We are wise to express our willingness for God to do whatever he wishes to do and to say whatever he wishes to say, even if it would seem he prefers to simply be *with* us without saying or doing anything in particular.

- Take the first twenty or thirty minutes to do nothing more than listen. Be quiet. Sit still or take an unhurried stroll. Notice God in the beauty of what he has made. Prayerfully enter God's presence as a listener rather than as a speaker. Listen with your ears, but also with your eyes, your mind, your heart.

- Give thanks. I have found that gratitude and thanksgiving are evidence of an unhurried life. When we are hurried, we often fail to take time to say a simple "thank you" to God, or anyone else for that matter. It takes time to notice the good and acknowledge it to God with gratitude.

- I find it helpful to become as quiet on the outside as I am able. In that place of outward silence, I become aware of the noise of my driven soul. The challenge at this point is whether I will stay with God, seeking to be still and silent in his presence, or allow the inner noise and drivenness to decide my next step. Of course it will be an action step! But if I linger with God, I begin to sense his love quieting my fear, his peace replacing my anxiety, his comfort touching my pain, his mercy forgiving my waywardness, his grace providing what I most need in the depths of my soul. When we are patient enough to wait in silence for the inner noise to weary of its aim to keep us moving, thinking and doing, we can then remember that he really *is* God.

- When distractions come—and they will—you might choose to just let them float by rather than wrestling with them. Or you might find a way to include those distractions in your time with the Lord: give thanks for them, make a request regarding them or entrust them into God's hands. I was at a retreat center once, looking for some time to be quiet and alone with God, when the gardener decided it was time to crank up the leaf blower right near where I was sitting. Talk about distraction! I felt frustrated. I wanted to go talk to him or to the retreat director about this thoughtless act. But I began to sense Jesus drawing me to give thanks for the gardener's care for this little piece of property. As I did this, my heart softened, and what had felt like a distraction from my time with God actually drew me closer to him.

A "ONE-THIRD" RULE

I've been in vocational Christian ministry for over thirty years. I've led a lot of events, gatherings, conferences, retreats, leadership team meetings and so on. As I have been leading such meetings more recently—and training others as they lead them—I've appreciated a guideline that my friend and colleague Paul Jensen recommends. He calls it the "One-Third Rule," and it's simple: however much time an event or series of events involves, we make one-third of those hours the actual practice of what we are training for, especially as it relates to communion with God and community with one another.[2] This principle keeps us from doing a lot of talking, teaching and training based on the assumption that participants will then go home and figure out on their own how to practice what we've preached.

Perhaps, like me, you have accumulated sermon notes, seminar notes, retreat notes or any number of other resources from one gathering or another, and this fine information has found its way onto a shelf or into a drawer, long forgotten, much less looked at. We've found that the One-Third Rule provides space for training a group to actually do instead of merely learning ideas. This unhurried approach may leave less time for teaching content, but what we do teach gets practiced and therefore actually learned rather than just thought about. This approach—an apprenticeship design—reflects the practice of Jesus when he was developing his disciples.

I often travel hundreds, even thousands of miles to be with a group of leaders to lead a retreat or do some training. The practical impulse in those who invite me to come is to pack every possible minute with training *about* various spiritual practices, theories or insights. I understand the rationale. We want to get as much good training as possible within a limited time and in view of the costs involved. I just want them to get it not only into their minds but into their hearts and their habits. And this happens when we try on what we're learning while we're together.

For example, I enjoy consulting ministries to help them plan retreats that will enable them to evaluate their organizational purposes and goals. In one case, the desired outcome of a particular retreat was a clear set of ministry goals for the coming year. Such planning times can be exciting, but also mind-numbing. They can be tense as many people share different opinions. Following the One-Third Rule, I take the first third of the retreat to guide participants in anything but the actual work we intend to accomplish by the end of our time together. Instead, I make space for spiritual practices like *lectio divina*, solitude and silence, and contemplative intercession as well as for communal practices like sharing with one another what God is doing in our lives, praying for one another, affirming one another and so on.

During a recent planning retreat I facilitated, we spent most of day one seeking God's presence, God's leadership and God's way *first*. We then invested day two in the creative group work of discerning goals for the coming year of ministry. In this particular case, the leadership team unexpectedly finished its work on day two an hour earlier than they had scheduled. Each one commented that, far from diminishing the quality and quantity of their strategic work (after all, they were spending less time on it), the many hours they had set aside for personal solitude, personal and group reflection on a couple of key passages, and communal prayer had actually multiplied the fruitfulness (both in quality and quantity) of their work beyond what they felt they would have produced if they had merely "opened in prayer" and spent two full days on the work. They were more unified, creative and energized as a result of how the retreat began with such unhurried time. And I am seeing this outcome over and over again.

Now this isn't to say that spiritual practices like solitude, silence, community, intercession or *lectio divina* should be used in a utilitarian manner. The One-Third Rule offers a simple application on an organizational level of Jesus' straightforward and powerful words: "Seek first his kingdom and his righteousness, and all these things will be given to you as well" (Mt 6:33). Of course, "all these things" in the original context is referring to food and clothing—basic needs—but it's no stretch to expect that we might count on our good God to pour out what an organization needs (such as wisdom, unity, creativity, insight, mutual care, emotional buoyancy and energy, to name a few) when we are doing ministry strategizing or program planning.

I am grateful that God is growing my confidence that this more unhurried approach proves far more fruitful than the hurried approach I've been accustomed to in the past. Taking a two-day planning retreat and devoting the first third of that time to an unhurried seeking of God himself in order to listen to him and respond to him produces fertile soil where good planning and strategizing can grow and bear fruit.

SLOWING

As our culture becomes more and more hurried, I am learning the value of the spiritual discipline of slowing. Toward that end, I do a little experiment from time to time: I sometimes drive in the slowest lane of traffic on the freeway. (In Southern California, though, just driving the freeway speed limit feels like slowing!) I try to pay attention to how I feel. Am I anxious? Frustrated? Irritable? Impatient? (What thoughts are going through your mind in this moment as you step into this scenario?) I try to determine what negative outcome I am so nervously anticipating and just how realistic that expectation is. How dire would such an outcome actually be—and why do I think that? I also ask myself what I'm going to do with the extra minutes I think I'm gaining by driving so fast. Besides, what kind of "me" will be arriving when I get to my destination a few minutes earlier? Will I be as able to represent Jesus as I would if I slowed down a bit and were more present in the moment on the way?

In a similar exercise, when I am walking, I sometimes choose to walk a bit more slowly. I try to rediscover the ancient art of strolling. Or when I'm writing an email, I may take a moment to thank the Lord for the person to whom I am writing, or I may ask him to guide my communication. This kind of slowing enriches the work I do as well as the person I am becoming—by God's gracious and transforming power.

Another way I practice slowing is by setting aside no- or low-tech times in my schedule. Perhaps like you, I almost always have a phone in my pocket, an iPad in my briefcase and a computer on my desk. This ever-present technology has a way of accelerating my inner life. My mobile phone makes me virtually omnipresent: I'm nearly *always* available. In an era far preceding mobile phones, Elton Trueblood warned about this: a person who is always available is not worth enough when they are available.[3]

This discipline is a hard one for me. I was the kid in high school who, as part of the school's math club (that bastion of coolness), helped solder together an Imsai 8080 processor that could only be programmed by flipping hexadecimal switches. I really like technology, but I wasn't created to serve it. Technology was developed to serve me, to paraphrase a familiar saying of Jesus about the

Sabbath (Mk 2:27). Technology is a means to many good ends, but it is not to be an end in itself.

Finally, another simple, though not easy, slowing practice that can help us unhurry our lives is to follow James's counsel: "Be quick to listen, slow to speak and slow to become angry" (Jas 1:19). In my conversations, however, I am often tempted to listen in order to formulate my next words rather than to truly hear and understand. Listening well is key—and I have so much to learn. In my seminary training, I took a number of classes on preaching and teaching where I learned how to speak well, but I don't remember receiving any training in how to listen. When I fail to listen well, I become a dispenser of quick, generic responses to people whose lives are unfamiliar to me. I may even have much experience to share, but I can't offer guidance if I don't know what a person is dealing with, what the feelings behind the words are. Furthermore, being quick to listen and slow to speak is made more of a challenge by our noisy and word-filled world. James's advice offers a wise and fruitful orientation for all of our relationships, our work and our lives.

Sleep

We are an increasingly sleep-deprived culture. The Centers for Disease Control and Prevention suggests that the average adult needs about seven to nine hours of sleep per night for good health, while a survey by the National Health Interview Survey in 2005–2007 found that nearly 30 percent of adults average less than six hours,[4] reflecting a drop in average sleep time of more than 20 percent over the last century.[5] Why aren't we getting enough sleep? At least one reason is our habit of burning the candle at both ends of our days: we get up early and we stay up late in our hurrying to get more and more done.

Douglas Steere, a Quaker professor writing at the midpoint of the last century, made this observation:

At few points do well-meaning persons violate training, reveal their lack of intentional living, and dissipate their energies more consistently than in the matter of sleep. Sufficient sleep and no more should be gotten so that the [person] feels rested and refreshed upon awakening. Nothing makes inward prayer more difficult than a consistently sleep-starved body.[6]

In the same way we look at other forms of rest, we are tempted to see sleep as a waste of our time, a break in the rhythm of our productivity. But what if sleep is one of God's gifts to us that we are failing to open? Of course we can sleep too much, but it is far more likely that many of us are not sleeping enough. Consider the ancient wisdom of the Rule of Benedict: "In his plan of life, Benedict set aside four hours a day for prayer, six to nine hours a day for work, seven to nine hours for sleep, about three hours for eating and rest, and three hours a day for reading and reflection time."[7]

Another way to open this gift of sleep is through the time-honored practice of taking a nap. When I took my training in spiritual direction at the Pecos Benedictine Abbey in 2000–2001, I got to know Father Sam. Before going to the Abbey, Father Sam had lived for forty years as a Trappist monk with a rigorous and austere cadence. He was still in the habit of rising at 2 a.m. even though others at Pecos did not observe that rhythm. As a result, Father Sam would find himself a bit tired midday after lunch. So he would often walk through the common area of the monastery and announce that he was getting ready to practice one of his favorite spiritual disciplines—*napcio divina*. We laughed, of course, but I have come to see the wisdom of welcoming God's gift of little rests in the midst of a busy day or busy season.

SEEKING GUIDANCE

When we ask God for guidance, many of us expect him to hand us a map. We want turn-by-turn directions to the place we are heading. That's what Google gives us! But have we asked whether where we are going is where he is going? Or are we asking him for directions to a place he isn't headed?

What if, instead of a road map, God is offering to be my guide? What if I let him decide where we are going? And what if I stopped demanding a lot of directions from him in advance and instead trusted him to guide my next turn once we are in the neighborhood? After all, God seems to prefer guiding us in a way that keeps us close to him—and his way of guiding us is unhurried. He would prefer to guide me as my companion for the journey rather than hand me directions that I'd be tempted to run off with, leaving him in the dust. Maybe I could learn to ask less for God's guidance and more for a sense that he is being my guide; to ask less for help and more for the awareness that he wants to be my helper; and to ask less for strength and more for confidence that he is my stronghold.

CONCLUSION

As you reflect back on the suggested practices of solitude and silence, Extended Personal Communion with God (EPC), unhurried leadership, slowing, sleep, slowness to speak or seeking guidance, which of these sounds the most challenging for you at this stage of your journey? Why? Which sounds most inviting? Which of the unhurrying practices I've mentioned in this chapter is God inviting you to practice now? My prayer is that you will choose one and do it as an offering to the unhurried Savior who longs to have you abide in him. When you've taken that little step, then take another. When you do so, you will have embarked on a more unhurried journey.

UNHURRIED TIME

1. As you think about steps you can take to unhurry your life,

what habits or practices are already helping you do so? What current habits or practices tend to accelerate your life?

2. When you review some of the practices mentioned in this chapter—solitude and silence (EPC), unhurried leadership, slowing, sleep, slowness to speak, seeking guidance—which one do you find most attractive? Why? Which seems most challenging? Why is that?

3. What next step related to one of these practices might God be inviting you to take? When do you think you'll take this step? Whom will you talk to about this so you can be encouraged and supported in prayer?

An Eternal Life

You've probably noticed that it's easier to be unhurried during some moments than it is during others. Recently, I found myself in the Dominican Republic leading one of our Journey retreats for pastors and other Christian leaders there. We were at a conference center, just outside the town of Jarabacoa, nestled up against the greenest, lushest mountains you can imagine. It felt like paradise. You would think this would be a place where living an unhurried life would be easy, if even for just the four days we were there. And there's truth to that assumption.

In this peaceful town, though, is a place called *La Confluencia*. It is the meeting point—the confluence—of two of the country's main rivers. When two rivers come together, the waters become tumultuous and turbulent, not unlike my life in this season— although I feel as if I'm experiencing the confluence of more than just two rivers! This has been one of my busiest seasons of ministry in recent memory, and at the same time, I am enjoying the blessing of a busier family with all three of my sons now teenagers. And against this backdrop are—of course!—some personal soul issues that have proven to be quite challenging, demanding much time and energy. Yet, in the midst of all this, God has helped me realize that if this idea of being unhurried is not helpful to me in the here and now, it probably won't be much help to anyone else either!

I'm also realizing that if an unhurried life is only possible when life is uneventful and undemanding, that kind of unhurry is not the fruit of following Jesus' rhythm of hard work *and* deep rest, of caring for the multitudes *and* being cared for by his Father. We read that early in Jesus' ministry "the news about him spread all the more, so that crowds of people came to hear him and to be healed of their sicknesses. But Jesus often withdrew to lonely places and prayed" (Lk 5:15-16). Jesus knew—and lived—an unhurried life in the face of lots of demands and many needy people. As we've seen, he invites you and me to an unhurried life that may actually be quite busy at times.

It's in these very busy seasons and stretches of my life and work that I can easily lose sight of the most unhurried reality of all—eternal life.

AN UNHURRIED ETERNITY

When you think about eternal life, what most excites you . . . or depresses you? What is your vision of eternal life? Is your vision nothing more than a blurry sense of being somewhere in God's neighborhood until the end of time and beyond? Or is eternal life merely a matter of unending duration? (I hope that many of my current activities and involvements won't last forever, but I can think of a few that I hope will.) Are you focused more on the *eternal* or on the *life*? Over time, I'm realizing that I would be very grateful for unending *life*. As in real life. Deep life. Joyful life.

When I first came to know Jesus and trust in him, my main idea of eternal life was one of negation: I was now no longer in danger of eternal punishment. I was told I'd spend forever with God after I died—which I assumed would be a good thing—but I had little sense of exactly what that meant for my future, let alone my present. Here's one possibility: if we have eternal life in Christ, then we have unlimited time. I'm not talking about a perspective that allows or encourages procrastination; I'm talking about the "eternal life" perspective that exposes the lie that "I just don't have time for this, that or the other." How many times do we say no to good things because of this mistaken belief that we don't have time? Every time I say the words "I don't have time," I am strengthening the hold that hurry has on me. The reality is that all of us on this planet have the same amount of time day by day, and, in Christ, we have all of eternity. Put differently, in Christ, I have all the time I need for whatever God is giving me to do or inviting me into. And that is an eternal-life—an unhurried-life—perspective.

Yet sometimes, as an encouragement to grab for all that life has to offer, we tell ourselves, *You only live once!* There is, of course, a great deal of truth in this. We may encounter certain opportunities only once, and our failure to respond may cost us profoundly. But from another perspective, if we're living an eternal life in Jesus, our "only live once" lasts forever. This viewpoint doesn't prevent us from taking risks, pushing through fears or seizing opportunities. Instead, this spacious perspective just might help us realize that we can anticipate many good occasions to grow, be stretched and make progress on our eternal path of transformation. We might, for instance, find courage to stay with a hard lesson until we learn it. We may realize that we have time to make the mistakes necessary for a life lesson to sink in and stick.

As far as an unhurried vision of life is concerned, I am coming to believe that eternal life is its ultimate expression. My tendency to live a far more hurried version of life, even of the Christian life, has had a way of constricting my perspective, diminishing my joy and driving me into the tyranny of the current task. And on top of whatever I'm working on now, I pile on the weight of all the tasks already on my plate, those tasks that seem to be waiting with little patience to become my current task. Kierkegaard said that "the press of busyness is like a charm. Its power swells. . . . It reaches out seeking always to lay hold of ever-younger victims so that childhood or youth are scarcely allowed the quiet and the retirement in which the Eternal may unfold a divine growth."[1] Busyness is very enticing, but I'm coming to believe that, for me, hurry squeezes the life out of the present moment.

So What *Is* Eternal Life?

The simplest and most straightforward answer I've found to the question "What is eternal life?" is found in the words Jesus spoke to his inner circle in the upper room on his last night with them. He spoke these words in prayer: "Now *this* is eternal life: that they know you, the only true God, and Jesus Christ, whom you have sent" (Jn 17:3, emphasis mine). Eternal life is not so much a matter of mere duration or a guarantee of a pleasant future. Eternal life is an ongoing relationship of mutual love with the One who *is* Life. It is a relationship I enjoy now and will enjoy into forever. My initial trust in Jesus has all of forever to grow into rich and full communion with the faithful One.

Eternal life is life in God. It is our ever-deepening, conversational relationship with the One who has proven his love for us beyond imagination. Eternal life is eternal *life*, eternal *living*. Eternal life is living with Father, Son and Spirit forever. Eternity is enough time to discover just how interesting, how intelligent, how capable, how enjoyable, how engaging Jesus really is. I'd use words like *glorious, wise, powerful, gracious* and *majestic*, but these adjectives have been somewhat emptied of meaning by overuse in religious circles. I know—and I am saddened—that I have lost much of my ability to regard these life-giving realities with faith, hope and gratitude.

Jesus closed his prayer to the Father with these words: "I have made you known to them, and will continue to make you known in order that the love you have for me may be in them and that I myself may be in them" (Jn 17:26). Jesus wants us to know the Father; in fact, he came to show us the Father (see Jn 14:7).

Knowing the Father

Just before a new school year began, I scheduled a three-day retreat in San Diego. I had a friend's home there, overlooking the Mission Valley area, all to myself. I was there, in part, to work on a course I would soon be teaching. But for two days I wrestled and struggled and produced nothing. I could not concentrate for the life of me! I felt distracted and uncreative. I went to bed that second night wondering if I'd have anything at all to show for these three days away.

At 3 a.m. on the morning of the third day, I awoke and could not go back to sleep. As I lay awake in bed, still feeling upset and disappointed about how unproductive the time had been, I found myself praying, "God, I need your help. I need you to meet me in this distracted and frustrating place."

As I lay there in the quiet, I became aware of a strong and alarming thought: *Right now, I don't feel very welcome or wanted in God's presence. How am I supposed to teach a class recommending him to others?* I realized that the God in my gut was very different from the God of my professed beliefs.

So I prayed, "Jesus, I need to see the Father more truly. I need to see him as he really is. There must be a distorted image of him somewhere in my heart and mind that I'm repelled by rather than drawn to."

Almost immediately, I heard in my heart the very similar words of Philip to Jesus in the upper room: "Lord, show us the Father and that will be enough for us" (Jn 14:8). Jesus opens Philip's eyes (and mine) in his answer to the request by saying, basically, "You've been with me for three years. You've watched how I've lived. You've seen what I've done. You've heard what I said. All of this has been the Father's nature on display. The Father is like me. I am like my Father. We are One. I haven't been living my life *for* the Father so much as *in* the Father, and he has lived in me all this time. Didn't you realize that? I speak with his authority. I live in his love and power.

"Now, Philip (and Alan), *this* is what I invited you into. Trust me. Believe in me when I say this. You've watched how I lived in the Father. Now I say to you, 'Live in the Father through me.' Let the Father work through you, speak through you, live in and through you. Just as the Father has shown himself in and through me, let him now do the same in and through you. Ask whatever you wish in this way. I want it. The Father wants it. And, deep down, you know that you want it as well."

I realized that my gut image of God was that of a rejecting father—a human father on a bad day—rather than the loving, joyful, gentle Father I see reflected in the face of Jesus. Of course I didn't want to be alone or quiet with the negative vision of God I had in my gut at that moment! *But*, my thoughts continued, *eternal life is* knowing *the Father—really knowing him as Jesus came to make him known. Nothing is more life-giving than this.*

So eternal life is unhurried life in relationship with our loving heavenly Father, and my present physical life offers only a glimpse of that forever life. Thomas Kelly, a Quaker author of the last century, put it this way:

> We no longer live merely in time but . . . also in the Eternal. The world of time is no longer the sole reality of which we are aware. A second Reality hovers, quickens, quivers, stirs, energizes us, breaks in upon us and in love embraces us, together with all things, within Himself. We live our lives at two levels simultaneously, the level of time and the level of

the Timeless. They form one sequence, with a fluctuating border between them.[2]

Are you and I learning to live in this dual awareness? Do we think of time and eternity as sequential—this and then that—or as concurrent? Does my life reflect my growing confidence in the truth that I will live forever? Or does my life look as though I believe the universe might come to an abrupt end if I don't keep moving? You and I are actually living eternal life now.

LIVING THIS UNHURRIED LIFE

Jesus said that eternal life is knowing the Father and knowing Jesus as the One sent by the Father. The writer of Hebrews invites us into this unhurried, eternal-life perspective:

> Since we are surrounded by such a great cloud of witnesses, let us throw off everything that hinders and the sin that so easily entangles. And let us run with perseverance the race marked out for us, fixing our eyes on Jesus, the pioneer and perfecter of faith. (12:1-2)

When I'm living my life always in the fast lane, I find it very hard to fix my eyes on Jesus—or on anything other than what's in the lane just ahead of me. But I have found that fixing the eyes of my heart on Jesus has a way of creating in me a holy slowing. My frantic, anxious way is decelerated as the Spirit helps me see Jesus more clearly wherever I am, whatever I'm doing. I am also learning from Jesus' own unhurried way how to live like he lived.

God himself extends this invitation to us through the apostle Paul:

> Since, then, you have been raised with Christ, set your hearts on things above, where Christ is, seated at the right hand of God. Set your minds on things above, not on earthly things.

For you died, and your life is now hidden with Christ in God. When Christ, who is your life, appears, then you also will appear with him in glory. (Col 3:1-4)

Having named Jesus as my Savior and Lord, I am risen with Christ, so the invitation to me is to set my heart and my mind on the risen One who is above, not on merely earthly things. When I am hurried, those earthly things seem to get all my attention. I lose sight of the real presence of Christ *with* me, the actual presence of Christ *in* me, the presence of the One seated in favor at the Father's right hand.

Now I would propose that "things above" versus "earthly things" may not be two different categories of things but perhaps two different perspectives on the *same* things. After all, it makes sense that I can only enjoy and fully enter into *anything* if I do so in Jesus, with my mind and heart resting and rooted in his presence, remembering and grounded in the reality that my life is eternal.

But—and I'm sure this is your experience too—it's hard to set my heart and mind on things above when I'm racing from earthly thing to earthly thing down here below. Yet with his invitation to us to "set our hearts" (Col 3:1) or "set our minds" (Col 3:2) on things above, I don't think the apostle Paul was saying, "Think constant God thoughts and feel constant God feelings." I believe Paul was saying something closer to "Live in the remembered and realized companionship of Christ." I'm invited to remember that Jesus is always with me and I am always with him. Something dramatic happens when I both trust him and entrust myself to him. The necessary death that results means the beginning of a real yet hidden life. To be specific, my life is not limited merely to the obvious realities of earth that surround me. At the same time, my life is also "hidden with Christ in God" (Col 3:3): I am living my life in relationship—in communion—with my Lord. I can learn to live my life on two planes at once.

Knowing in my mind that Christ *is* my life—that I am alive with Jesus and in him—and wanting to live in that reality, I find myself praying, "Father, may your Spirit enable me to know vital communion with you from day to day."

One more note. I often say to leaders I meet with in spiritual direction that anything worth doing is worth starting small. That truth is relevant to our desire to cultivate an awareness of God's constant presence with us and around us. Many of us have a tendency to start heroically, but we grow tired or overwhelmed and we give up the effort. Starting small is like planting a seed, watering it day by day until it grows, tending to it well until it bears fruit. This "start small" approach is not as dramatic as the heroics, but it's far more fruitful in the long run.

FREEDOM AND SPACE

Another important truth—stated here by the apostle Paul—encourages me to live an unhurried life. Let's learn from Paul's experience:

> Where the Spirit of the Lord is, there is freedom. And we all, who with unveiled faces contemplate the Lord's glory, are being transformed into his image with ever-increasing glory, which comes from the Lord, who is the Spirit. (2 Cor 3:17-18)

I have found—as you may have—that hurry becomes a veil that obscures the Lord's grandeur and beauty. Then, because my vision of his glory is hazy, my experience of transformation is hindered. Oh, I have engaged in spiritual practices, but I've done so behind the veil of hurry. As a result, instead of seeing the glory of the Lord and being transformed over time by such a vision, I have actually hidden my face in my spiritual practices. A veil of hurriedness, fueled by a sense of drivenness, keeps me from beholding the Almighty's face.

I have found guidance for contemplating the Lord's glory—once I slow down—in Richard Rohr's *The Naked Now*. Although we come from different theological neighborhoods of the church, I find a meeting place with him in Jesus. At one point, Rohr uses a number of phrases to describe the nature of contemplation, of staying spiritually awake. (His phrases appear in italics below.)[3]

"I drop to a level deeper than the passing show." We're tempted to call that "passing show" *real* life, but it isn't really. All of the megaconcerns on the surface level are insignificant in light of the eternal reality God's people know. Some things that have me incredibly worried here and now would not even register in my consciousness if I were more aware of the Father's eternal kingdom. To gain that awareness—to be able to live my life on two planes—I can choose to deal with the realities at hand with continual prayer, with a mind and heart set on higher things, with an eternal perspective.

"I become the calm seer of my dramas from that level." Some of these descriptions sound like the work I've done in therapy where I recognize some of the childish and adolescent emotions within me, becoming separate enough from them to discern them and choose, instead, to live from a mature, adult perspective. I can experience a peace that does not reflect the stir of the surface, but comes from a deeper place.

"I watch myself compassionately from a little distance, almost as if the 'myself' is someone else—'a corpse,' as St. Francis put it." To "watch myself compassionately from a little distance" sounds so inviting. It would be dying to the "me" that has been misshapen in this God-disregarding world. I would learn to live less on autopilot. I would learn to care for those immature parts of myself that are anxious and fearful about life. I would make some space within where I could receive God's affection and take it deeply in.

"I dis-identify with my own emotional noise, and no longer let it pull me here and there, up and down." My feelings, though real,

aren't to be my primary reality. My feelings are noisy, they are demanding, they are pushy—but they aren't the last word. I need not be trapped in emotional noise. I don't need to try to escape from my emotions or numb myself to them, but I can stop handing the reins of my life over to them. I can choose instead to live my life under the mighty yet gentle reign of Christ. What if I were able to live out the truth that the emotional noise is not the greatest reality of my life and, in fact, may not be much of a reality at all?

The apostle Paul wrote about the essential reality of our life on this planet:

> Though outwardly we are wasting away, yet inwardly we are being renewed day by day. For our light and momentary troubles are achieving for us an eternal glory that far outweighs them all. So we fix our eyes not on what is seen, but on what is unseen, since what is seen is temporary, but what is unseen is eternal. (2 Cor 4:16-18)

I find a prayer rising up in response to this passage: "Enable me, Lord, to be far less focused on the outward withering and more trusting of the hidden but unshakable reality of daily inward renewal. Help me remember that if I'm being renewed, it's not my doing but yours. I don't always feel that renewal happening, but I do trust you to be the renewer of my life.

"And, Father, I have to say that my troubles don't ever feel light and momentary when I fail to see them in light of your presence with me. They are only light compared to the weighty glory that lies ahead. They are only momentary compared to eternity. I need to live with this perspective, Lord, so help me learn how to do what seems impossible to me: help me learn to gaze at the unseen eternal. It's so much easier to stare at my visible troubles than to learn to fix my attention on the renewing work of the Spirit that I don't readily perceive."

Unhurried Communion with Jesus

If you have read to this point, you don't need me to remind you that I didn't write this book so that more people will live a life of leisure. That's not at all the kind of unhurry I've had in mind. Instead, I am hungry to be part of a community of men and women who are living more fully and deeply in unhurried communion with Jesus, who are walking with him, serving him and working with him. How rich such a life would be—not only for us but for the people around us. In fact, life lived in unhurried communion with the Almighty might invite his kingdom to come and his will to be done here among us just as it is being done in his presence. I also believe that our unhurried communion with our Shepherd will bear much fruit and will tantalize many to come to him, get to know him and choose to follow him.

I close this chapter—and this book—with a prayer:

Father, Son, Spirit,
enable us to live unhurried,
resting and communing with you.
Enlighten our eyes to see
whatever your Spirit is showing us.
Open our ears to hear
whatever your Spirit is saying to us.
Quiet our hearts
with your songs of love.
Draw our minds to focus on things above,
and not on empty human concerns.
May that which blesses us,
become a blessing to others.
We ask this in the name of the Father,
and of the Son
and of the Holy Spirit. Amen.[4]

UNHURRIED TIME

1. What situations or circumstances in your life now contribute
   most to your sense of hurry? Take five or ten minutes to consider
   those situations and circumstances from the perspective of
   eternity. In what ways, if any, does this perspective help you?
   Now, can you imagine yourself in the unhurried presence of God
   despite these situations and circumstances? Why or why not?

2. What was your initial response to the idea that eternal life is
   unhurried? What conflict or tension, if any, does the idea of an
   unhurried eternal life prompt in you?

3. In what arenas of your life do you find it easiest to fix your eyes
   on Jesus, to set your heart and your mind on things above? In
   what arenas do you find it most difficult to fix your eyes on
   Jesus? Take a few minutes right now to talk with God about
   both these blessings and these challenges.

ACKNOWLEDGMENTS

When a book represents the insights and experiences of half a lifetime, how can an author express thanks to each one who made a difference along the way? Let me acknowledge a few who have been with me and have helped in my journey toward a more unhurried way of life and work.

I thank my colleagues at The Leadership Institute, especially the four who served as its founders in 1989: Paul Jensen, Chuck Miller, Jon Byron and Wayne Anderson (who departed for the unhurry of eternity in 2008). You have been dear brothers, fellow workers in ministry and fellow soldiers in prayer for nearly twenty-five years. Hardly a thought I think or a word I say is untouched by your influence. I'm also grateful for the rest of our staff and board: Joy, Craig, Wil, Chris, David, Jon and Lisa, Wendy, Joan, Don, Gary J., Sandy, and Gary T.

I owe a great debt of gratitude to hundreds of alumni from now over twenty generations who have participated in The Journey to Reach the Next Generations. What a gift to share this unhurried journey with you! Many of these chapters had their genesis as presentations in this spiritual leadership training process.

This book would not exist without the help and encouragement of Lisa Guest, who helped me believe I could write it and reviewed the earliest draft of this material. Jan Johnson served as my unofficial agent, opening the door for a first-time author to be published by what has long been my favorite publisher, InterVarsity Press. Cindy Bunch gave much-needed direction and help from start to finish. Many other friends reviewed and commented on early drafts and encouraged me in the project: Tom and Marla, Jeff and Mary, Graeme and Diane, Doug and Sabrina. Luz, a wonderful matriarch of the church in Santiago, Dominican Republic, prayed me out of a serious case of writer's block on the week my first draft was due.

In the midst of the writing journey, I began to live life together with a small but significant community of fellow Jesus-followers called, appropriately, The Following. I'm grateful to be learning this unhurried life with Jesus together with fellow lead-followers Doug Webster, Doug Fields, Tim Timmons, Charlie Koeller, Sherri Alden and Seth Bartlette.

Finally, I'm grateful for my best friend in the unhurried way, my wife of twenty-eight years, Gem. Your name has always described you so well. So much of what I've learned about the unhurried ways of Jesus, I've witnessed in you. Thank you for your great patience as I wrestle with (and stumble at) living what I write. I'm also grateful for my three sons, Sean, Bryan and Christopher, and the ways their generation is learning to be so much less hurried in life than mine has been. I'm proud of each of you. May the Lord be with you.

Notes

Chapter 1: A Frenetic Life

[1]John Ortberg, *The Life You've Always Wanted* (Grand Rapids: Zondervan, 1997), p. 81. Ortberg uses this advice as the introduction to chapter 5, "An Unhurried Life: The Practice of Slowing."

[2]Ibid., p. 84.

[3]You can read more about Bill's conversation with Dallas Willard at www .soulshepherding.org/articles/overcoming-problems/one-word/.

[4]See further in Paul Jensen, *Subversive Spirituality: Transforming Mission Through the Collapse of Space and Time* (Eugene, OR: Pickwick, 2009), pp. 62-65.

[5]Percy C. Ainsworth, "Faith and Haste," *Weavings*, January/February 2003, p. 11.

[6]Ronald Boyd-MacMillan, *Faith That Endures* (Grand Rapids: Revell, 2006), pp. 306-9.

[7]Ibid., p. 307.

[8]Ibid., p. 308.

[9]Peter Craigie's commentary translation—in *Psalms 1–50*, Word Biblical Commentary (Waco, TX: Word, 1983), p. 342—offers "Relax, and know that I am God" for Psalm 46:10.

[10]Wayne Muller, *Sabbath* (New York: Bantam Books, 1999), p. 70.

[11]J. B. Phillips, *Your God Is Too Small* (New York: Macmillan, 1961), pp. 55-56.

Chapter 2: An Unhurried Apprentice

[1]Elton Trueblood, "The Problem of the Crowd," in *The Yoke of Christ and Other Sermons* (New York: Harper & Brothers, 1958), pp. 110-11.

[2]Paul Jensen, *Subversive Spirituality: Transforming Mission Through the Collapse of Space and Time* (Eugene, OR: Pickwick, 2009), pp. 107-8.

[3]Dallas Willard, *The Great Omission* (New York: HarperCollins, 2006), p. 44.

Chapter 3: Productivity

[1]Gerald May, *The Awakened Heart* (San Francisco: HarperSanFrancisco, 1991), pp. 94-95.

[2]Brenda Ueland, *If You Want to Write* (Saint Paul, MN: Graywolf Press, 1938, 1987), p. 33.

[3]Kathleen Norris, *Acedia and Me* (New York: Riverhead Books, 2008), p. 3.

[4]Quoted in Columba Stewart, *Prayer and Community: The Benedictine Tradition* (Maryknoll, NY: Orbis Books, 1998), p. 76.

[5]Ibid., p. 77.

[6]Carl Honoré, *In Praise of Slowness* (San Francisco: HarperSanFrancisco, 2004), pp. 209-10.

[7]Quoted in Norris, *Acedia and Me,* pp. 130-31.

[8]John Ortberg, *The Life You've Always Wanted* (Grand Rapids: Zondervan, 1997), p. 78.

[9]Henri Nouwen, *The Way of the Heart* (New York: Harper & Row, 1981), p. 63.

[10]Joshua Choonmin Kang, *Deep-Rooted in Christ* (Downers Grove, IL: InterVarsity Press, 2007), p. 101.

[11]May, *Awakened Heart,* pp. 94-95.

[12]Thomas Merton, *The Last of the Fathers* (New York: Harcourt Brace Jovanovich, 1954), p. 60.

[13]Thomas Merton, *New Seeds of Contemplation* (New York: New Directions, 1961), pp. 206-7.

[14]Fr. Jean Baptiste Saint-Jure and Claude de la Colombiere, S.J., *Trustful Surrender to Divine Providence* (Charlotte, NC: TAN Books, 1983), pp. 77-78.

CHAPTER 4: TEMPTATION

[1]Kosuke Koyama, *Three Mile an Hour God* (Maryknoll, NY: Orbis, 1979), p. 3.

[2]Ronald Boyd-MacMillan, *Faith That Endures* (Grand Rapids: Revell, 2006), p. 6.

[3]Shirley Carter Hughson, *The Spiritual Letters of Shirley Carter Hughson* (West Park, NY: Holy Cross Press, 1953), p. 34.

[4]Henri Nouwen, *In the Name of Jesus* (New York: Crossroad, 1991), p. 38.

CHAPTER 5: UNHURRIED ENOUGH TO CARE

[1]Quoted in Eugene Peterson, *Tell It Slant* (Grand Rapids: Eerdmans, 2008), p. 72.

[2]Kosuke Koyama, *Three Mile an Hour God* (Maryknoll, NY: Orbis, 1979), p. 7.

[3]Ibid., p. 35.

[4]Quoted in Mark Buchanan, *The Rest of God: Restoring Your Soul by Restoring Sabbath* (Nashville: W Publishing Group, 2006), p. 79.

[5]Gerald May, *The Awakened Heart* (San Francisco: HarperSanFrancisco, 1991), p. 4.

[6]Cecile Andrews, *Slow Is Beautiful* (Gabriola Island, BC: New Society Publishers, 2006), p. 79.

[7]May, *Awakened Heart*, p. 78.

[8]Paul Jensen, *Subversive Spirituality* (Eugene, OR: Pickwick, 2009), p. 63. Jensen is quoting from D. K. Ulmer and L. Schwartzburd, "Treatment of Time Pathologies," *Heart and Mind: The Practice of Cardiac Psychology*, ed. Robert Allan and Stephen Scheidt (Washington, DC: American Psychological Association, 1996), p. 331.

[9]Paul Jensen, *Subversive Spirituality* (Eugene, OR: Pickwick, 2009), p. 64. Jensen is quoting from D. K. Ulmer and L. Schwartzburd, "Treatment of Time Pathologies," *Heart and Mind: The Practice of Cardiac Psychology*, ed. Robert Allan and Stephen Scheidt (Washington, DC: American Psychological Association, 1996), p. 331.

CHAPTER 6: UNHURRIED ENOUGH TO PRAY

[1]W. F. Adams, *Thoughts from the Note-Books of a Priest Religious* (Westminster: Faith Press, 1949), p. 7.

[2]Henri Nouwen, *Spiritual Formation* (New York: HarperOne, 2010), p. 20.

[3]E. Glenn Hinson, *Spiritual Preparation for Christian Leadership* (Nashville: Upper Room, 1999), p. 85.

[4]Frank Laubach, *Letters by a Modern Mystic* (Westwood, NJ: Fleming H. Revell, 1937, 1958), p. 56.

CHAPTER 7: REST

[1]Eugene Peterson, *Working the Angles* (Grand Rapids: Eerdmans, 1987), pp. 68-69.

[2]Abraham Heschel, *The Sabbath* (New York: Farrar, Strauss & Young, 1951), p. 14.

[3]This tendency is seen in Americans' vacationitis, failing to use about one-fifth of their paid time off. Carl Honoré, *In Praise of Slowness* (San Francisco: HarperSanFrancisco, 2004), pp. 5-6.

[4]Gerald May, *The Awakened Heart* (San Francisco: HarperSanFrancisco, 1991), p. 95.

[5]Allen Johnson, "In Search of the Affluent Society," *Human Nature* (September 1978): 50-59, in Robert Levine, *A Geography of Time: The Temporal Misadventures of a Social Psychologist* (New York: BasicBooks, 1997), pp. 13-14.

[6]Mark Buchanan, *The Rest of God: Restoring Your Soul by Restoring Sabbath* (Nashville: W Publishing Group, 2006), p. 98.

[7]Henri Nouwen, *Spiritual Direction* (San Francisco: HarperSanFrancisco, 2006), pp. 28-29.

[8]Tilden Edwards, *Sabbath Time* (Nashville: Upper Room, 1992), p. 15.

[9]Ibid., p. 13.

[10]Surveys have shown that mild depression is a common feeling after watching television sitcoms. Martin Seligman, *Authentic Happiness* (New York: Free Press, 2004), p. 117.

[11]Joan Chittister, OSB, *Wisdom Distilled from the Daily* (New York: Harper-Collins, 1990), p. 97.

[12]Ibid., p. 100.

[13]Stuart Brown, *Play* (New York: Penguin, 2009), p. 17.

[14]Wayne Muller, *Sabbath: Finding Rest, Renewal, and Delight in Our Busy Lives* (New York: Bantam Books, 1999), pp. 82-83.

[15]Thomas Merton, *No Man Is an Island* (New York: Harcourt Brace & Company, 1955), p. 123.

[16]See Amos 8:4-6; 2 Kings 4:23; Isaiah 66:23.

Chapter 8: Suffering

[1]J. B. Phillips, *Your God Is Too Small* (New York: Macmillan, 1961), p. 7.

[2]This introduction first appeared on the *Conversations Journal* blog on November 30, 2011, http://conversationsjournal.com/2011/11/pain-slows-us-down/.

[3]John of the Cross, "The Dark Night," *John of the Cross: Selected Writings*, ed. Kieran Kavanaugh (New York: Paulist Press, 1987), p. 186 (book one, ch. 10.5).

[4]F. B. Meyer, *The Secret of Guidance* (Chicago: Moody Press, n.d.), p. 80, emphasis in original.

Chapter 9: Maturity

[1]Eugene Peterson, *Practice Resurrection* (Grand Rapids: Eerdmans, 2010), p. 133.

[2]Brother Lawrence, *The Practice of the Presence of God,* trans. Salvatore Sciurba, OCD (Washington, DC: ICS Publications, 1994), p. 67.

[3]Baron Friedrich von Hügel, *Selected Letters 1896–1924,* ed. Bernard Holland (London: J. M. Dent & Sons, 1927), p. 266.

[4]Paul E. Hersey and Kenneth Blanchard, *Management of Organizational Behavior: Utilizing Human Resources,* 5th ed. (Englewood Cliffs, NJ: Prentice Hall, 1988), p. 4, emphasis mine.

[5]Shirley Carter Hughson, *The Spiritual Letters of Shirley Carter Hughson* (West Park, NY: Holy Cross Press, 1953), pp. 212-13.

[6]Peterson, *Practice Resurrection,* p. 7.

[7]I think of the story told in Kent Carlson and Mike Lueken's book, *Renovation of the Church* (Downers Grove, IL: InterVarsity Press, 2011), as a powerful example of just such an experiment.

[8]Thomas Kelly, *A Testament of Devotion* (New York: Harper & Brothers, 1941), pp. 36-37.

[9]Peterson, *Practice Resurrection,* pp. 222-23.

CHAPTER 10: SPIRITUAL PRACTICES FOR UNHURRYING

[1]Elton Trueblood, *The Company of the Committed* (New York: Harper & Row, 1961), pp. 43-44.

[2]Paul Jensen, *Subversive Spirituality* (Eugene, OR: Pickwick, 2009), p. 286.

[3]Trueblood, *The Company of the Committed,* p. 44.

[4]See "Insufficient Sleep Is a Public Health Epidemic," Centers for Disease Control and Prevention, March 17, 2011, www.cdc.gov/Features/dsSleep/.

[5]James Gleick, *Faster: The Acceleration of Just About Everything* (New York: Pantheon Books, 1999), p. 122.

[6]Douglas V. Steere, *Time to Spare* (New York: Harper & Brothers, 1949), p. 78.

[7]Joan Chittister, OSB, *Wisdom Distilled from the Daily* (New York: HarperCollins, 1990), pp. 98-99.

CHAPTER 11: AN ETERNAL LIFE

[1]Søren Kierkegaard, *Purity of Heart Is to Will One Thing* (New York: Harper & Row, 1956), p. 107, in John Ortberg, *The Life You've Always Wanted* (Grand Rapids: Zondervan, 1997), p. 91.

[2]Thomas Kelly, *A Testament of Devotion* (New York: Harper & Brothers, 1941), pp. 55-56.

[3]Richard Rohr, *The Naked Now* (New York: Crossroad, 2009), p. 135.

[4]Paraphrased from Ephesians 1:18; Revelation 2:7; Zephaniah 3:17; Colossians 3:2; and Genesis 12:2.

ALSO AVAILABLE

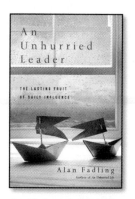

An Unhurried Leader
978-0-8308-4634-4

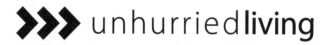 unhurried**living**

Many leaders feel hurried, and hurry is costing them more than they realize. Unhurried Living, founded by Alan and Gem Fadling, provides resources and training to help people learn to lead from fullness rather than leading on empty.

Great leadership begins on the inside, in your soul. Learning healthy patterns of rest and work can transform your leadership—your daily influence.

Built on more than twenty-five years of experience at the intersection of spiritual formation and leadership development, Unhurried Living seeks to inspire Christian leaders around the world to rest deeper so they can live fuller and lead better.

We seek to respond to questions many are asking:

Rest deeper. Why do I so often feel more drained than energized? Can I find space for my soul to breathe?

Live fuller. I have tried to fill my life with achievements, possessions, and notoriety, and I feel emptier than ever. Where can I find fullness that lasts?

Lead better. How can I step off the treadmill of mere busyness and make real, meaningful progress in my life and work?

Our purpose is to resource busy people so they can rediscover the genius of Jesus' unhurried way of life and leadership. We do this by . . .

Living all that we are learning so we share with others from experience and wisdom.

Developing digital, print, and video content that encourages the practices of an unhurried life.

Training people in Jesus' unhurried way of living and leading.

Come visit us at unhurriedliving.com to discover free resources to help you

Rest deeper. Live fuller. Lead better.

Web: unhurriedliving.com
Facebook: facebook.com/unhurriedliving
Twitter: @UnhurriedLiving
Instagram: UnhurriedLiving
Email: info@unhurriedliving.com